ISSUES IN SOCIETY

Are Mobile Devices Harmful?

Susan Henneberg

ReferencePoint Press®

San Diego, CA

About the Author

Susan Henneberg is the author of numerous children's and young adult nonfiction books. She lives and teaches in Reno, Nevada.

For more information, contact:
ReferencePoint Press, Inc.
PO Box 27779
San Diego, CA 92198
www. ReferencePointPress.com

LIBRARY OF CONGRESS CATALOGING-IN-PUBLICATION DATA

Names: Henneberg, Susan, author.
Title: Are mobile devices harmful? / by Susan Henneberg.
Description: San Diego, CA : ReferencePoint Press, Inc., 2017. | Series: Issues in society series | Audience: Grade 9 to 12. | Includes bibliographical references and index.
Identifiers: LCCN 2016016746 (print) | LCCN 2016020846 (ebook) | ISBN 9781682820964 (hardback) | ISBN 9781682820988 (eBook)
Subjects: LCSH: Cell phones--Health aspects--Juvenile literature.
Classification: LCC RA569.3 .H46 2017 (print) | LCC RA569.3 (ebook) | DDC 612/.014482--dc23
LC record available at https://lccn.loc.gov/2016016746

CONTENTS

A Deadly Crash

On a rainy September morning in 2006, nineteen-year-old Reggie Shaw was driving his Chevy sport-utility vehicle to work on a scenic Utah mountain highway. According to the driver of a pickup truck following at a distance, Shaw's vehicle wove back and forth across the center divide into the oncoming lane. During one fateful slip over the line, Shaw's SUV sideswiped a Saturn sedan carrying driver James Furfaro and his passenger, Keith O'Dell. These two individuals were scientists, husbands, and fathers. The impact spun their car sideways into Shaw's lane, and the trailing pickup truck plowed into the side of the Saturn, killing both men instantly. After authorities arrived, Shaw said he could not remember anything about the accident. "I crossed the center line, just a little bit, and I hit the car,"[1] he later told a counselor hired to help him process the event. When asked by police if he had been texting during that time, he said no. His cell phone records, however, told a different story.

Texting while driving was not against the law in Utah, or anywhere else, in 2006. This was an era of flip phones, and for many mobile phone users it was easier to make a call than laboriously tap out a text. Like many teens, though, Shaw had a lot of texting practice. He texted all day to keep in touch with friends and family. On that September morning, Shaw was planning to meet with his girlfriend later that evening. Records subpoenaed from his cell phone carrier showed ten minutes of back-and-forth texting near the time of the accident. The police detective who investigated the case did not believe that Shaw could not recall hitting the car.

Texting Puts Your Mind Somewhere Else

Also in 2006, a neuroscientist in San Francisco was asking what happens inside the brain when a person tries to do two things at once, or multitask. Dr. Adam Gazzaley's research was beginning to show a lot about the mind's ability to pay attention.

In particular, he wanted to know the effects of distraction on a person's attempts to focus on tasks. He amassed an array of brain imaging devices in his research lab: magnetic resonance imaging, positron-emission tomography scans, and electroencephalograms. He put students in front of driving simulators and sent texts to them while scanning their brains. His conclusion: "The eyes are open but the brain's not processing all the information."[2] To Gazzaley, Shaw might not have realized he hit the scientists' car because texting put his mind somewhere else.

> **"The eyes are open but the brain's not processing all the information."[2]**
>
> —Dr. Adam Gazzaley is director of the Cognitive Neuroscience Research Lab at the University of California–San Francisco.

The Utah prosecutors painstakingly built a case against Shaw, charging him with negligent homicide, a misdemeanor. Once Shaw saw the phone company records, he pleaded guilty to all charges against him, acknowledging that texting while driving caused the deadly crash. "This accident has affected my life forever," he told the court. "I can't even put it into words. And to see a law passed that would prevent people [from texting while driving] would mean a lot to me, to be able to know that nobody else would have to go through what I've gone through. That they would be aware of the dangers that this text messaging is, and what it can do, and the effects it can have."[3] Shaw served a sentence of eighteen days in jail and did community service. Part of his sentence mandated that he reach out to teens and educate them on the dangers of texting while driving. In 2007 Utah became the first state to pass laws specifically banning texting while driving.

The world has changed since Shaw's accident in 2006. Mobile technology has sparked a digital revolution around the world. Sophisticated and powerful gadgets provide information, education, and entertainment to billions of people, connecting and transforming the globe in ways scientists are only beginning to understand. To some observers, American teens use their smartphones the way they breathe: continuously and unconsciously. And it is not just teens who are riveted by what is on their mobile screens. Recent studies have shown that infants as young

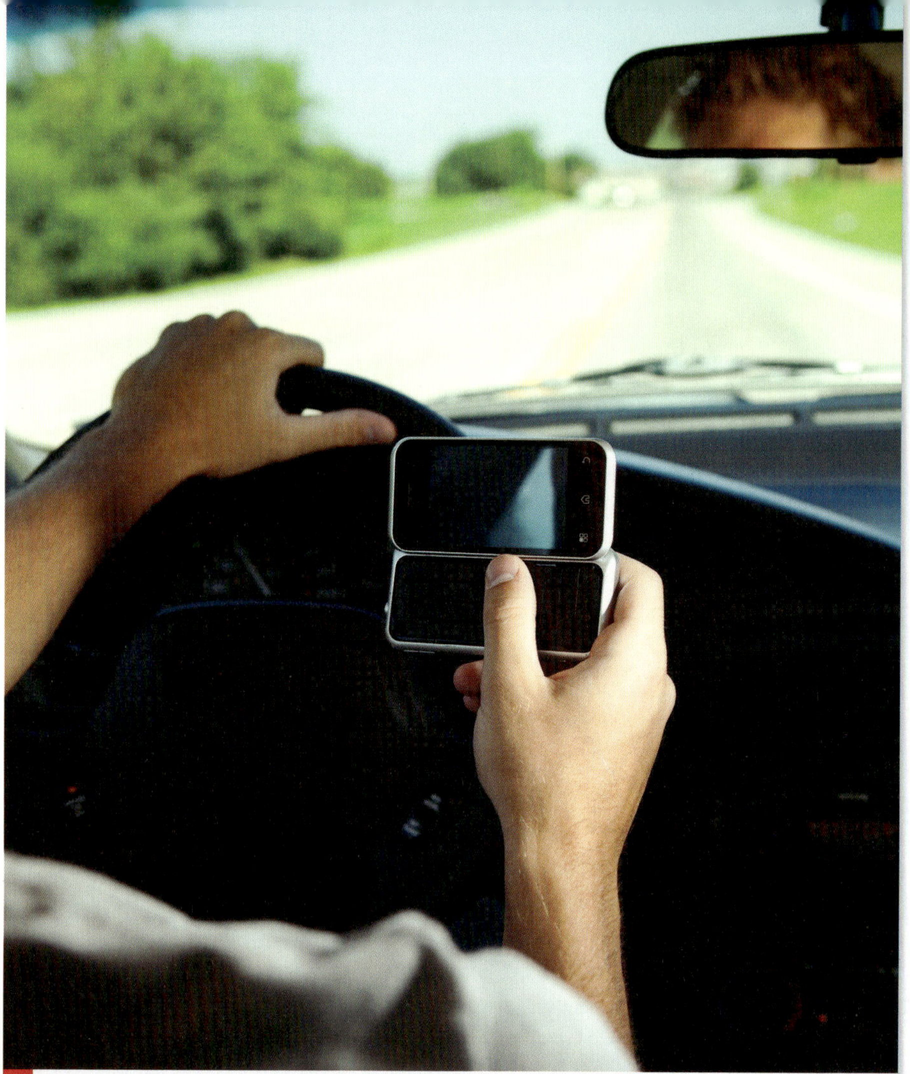

Despite the risks and illegality of texting while driving, many people continue to do it. Studies have shown that the danger arises because texting distracts a person's mind from the primary task of driving.

as twelve months can and do access media on smartphones. A 2015 study in *Pediatrics* showed that nearly 97 percent of American parents said their children used mobile devices of some sort, many while still infants. As much as mobile devices are impacting people's daily lives, they are also transforming their brains.

The Impact of Mobile Devices

Mobile phones, once brick-sized luxury items, have become extensions of the human body. What is the impact of mobile devices on the people who use them? Most people, especially teens and young adults, look positively upon their phones. More than 70 percent of phone users in one survey say that their mobile devices represent freedom and provide connection. Certainly phones have improved lives. Stories from developing countries show the impact phones have made just in the past ten years in public health, education, and access to information. Phones have improved work productivity, health, education, and daily life for some. They provide entertainment, escape, and relief from stress and boredom for others.

"To see a law passed that would prevent people [from texting while driving] would mean a lot to me, to be able to know that nobody else would have to go through what I've gone through."[3]

—Reggie Shaw was sentenced to jail for negligent homicide.

Regardless of the benefits, some observers fear that mobile devices might present users with unwanted consequences that may prove dangerous or, in Shaw's case, fatal. Mobile phones emit electromagnetic radiation, the effect of which is unknown. The words *compulsion* and *addiction* come up when people talk about the inability to turn off their devices. Some researchers argue that mobile phones interfere with sleep as well as study and work habits. Users complain that push notifications interrupt thinking and constant multitasking ruins the capacity for concentration. Texting has replaced face-to-face conversation for many people, and some experts worry that teens, who are the heaviest texters, are losing social skills, including the ability to empathize with others.

Like any other innovative technology, mobile devices affect users in unforeseen ways. Some commentators warn that mobile device owners need to use these powerful gadgets with awareness of their capabilities and knowledge of their drawbacks. Fatal collisions while driving and texting are only one tragic outcome that can happen to an unaware user. Those concerned argue that becoming educated about the potentially harmful impacts of mobile technology might help prevent more.

CHAPTER 1 What Are the Facts?

A 2014 headline in the British newspaper the *Independent* made a startling announcement: "There are officially more mobile devices in the world than people." Mobile phones, tablet computers, e-book readers, iPods, and handheld gaming devices are rapidly becoming essential gear for students, professionals, parents, and everyone else. These gadgets are multiplying five times faster than the population. The mobile phone leads the way. "No other technology has impacted us like the mobile phone," says Kevin Kimberlin, a technology expert. "It's the fastest growing manmade phenomenon ever—from zero to 7.2 billion in three decades."[4]

One accelerator of this growth is the change in the way people connect to the Internet. Once, the Internet was mainly accessed through desktop and laptop computers; now people access the Internet more often on mobile devices. According to a Pew Research Center 2015 survey, American media users, for example, spent 51 percent of their screen time on mobile devices, compared to 42 percent of screen time on desktop computers. Mobile phones and tablets live in purses, backpacks, and back pockets. They are always available for checking in with the office, connecting with friends and family, watching a video while waiting for a bus, shopping online, or planning a homework project. This ease of access to the Internet has transformed the way Americans work, drive, maintain social connections, and spend leisure time, experts say.

The World Is Connected

People around the globe have joined the revolution in mobile technology. As the world's most populous country, China leads the world in mobile device accounts, with more than 1.27 billion in 2014. Americans rank first, however, in the number of mobile devices per person. They have 103 mobile devices for every 100 citizens. The Chinese have 93 mobile devices for every 100 persons. India follows with 77 for every 100 persons. Other countries in Europe, Asia, North America, and South America are gaining rapidly. Most countries in Africa skipped the desktop and laptop era and moved directly into mobile connection.

Ownership of mobile devices is tied to level of income. Wealthier countries show the largest gains in mobile device usage. America, the wealthiest of countries, has embraced a variety of mobile technologies. Statistics collected by the Pew Research Center show just how connected Americans are. In 2014, 90 percent of adults in the United States owned a mobile phone. More than a third read books on an e-reader. Forty-two percent accessed social media and other applications, or apps, on a tablet.

> **"No other technology has impacted us like the mobile phone. It's the fastest growing manmade phenomenon ever—from zero to 7.2 billion in three decades."[4]**
>
> —Kevin Kimberlin is chair of the investment company Spencer Trask & Co.

Engaging with social media is the most popular use of mobile phones for those who can access the Internet through their phone. Mobile device users around the world use Facebook to stay in touch with family and friends and share their views on popular culture, religion, and politics. However, mobile devices also help users engage in other types of interpersonal transactions. For example, an important use for cell phones in East Africa is making or receiving mobile payments. Because banking is uncommon and often reserved for the wealthy, mobile carriers stepped in with a popular and widely used mobile money transfer and banking application.

Texting Is a Popular Way to Communicate

Almost all mobile phone owners use their devices for a lot more than making or receiving phone calls. For example, according to a Pew Research Center 2015 survey, 81 percent of Americans sent or received text messages. The lowest rate—35 percent—of texting among cell phone users was among those aged sixty-five or older. On average, this age group sent fewer than ten texts per day. In contrast to older cell phone users, 97 percent of teens texted. Most teens are master texters. Their average number of texts sent each day in America rose from 60 in 2009 to 167 in

2015. The survey notes that there is a gender gap in the rate of texting. Girls text twice as much as boys. The Pew teen survey showed that girls have long text exchanges with friends, check in with friends and family members to say hello several times a day, and text about school work. They use many abbreviations, punctuation marks, and emojis to add personality to their texts. Boys tend to use texting to respond to texts or arrange social engagements. Their texts are shorter and use fewer abbreviations and emojis. Boys also take longer to reply to texts than do girls.

The Pew survey found that one-third of teens with cell phones use text messaging apps such as WhatsApp, Kik Messenger, or iMessage. The highest use of these free apps is among Latino or African American teens and users at the lower end of the income spectrum. Because many users want their texts to be temporary,

The texting app WhatsApp (pictured) is one of several that are popular with teens. Such apps provide unlimited texting and do not deplete the usage limits on many users' cell phone plans.

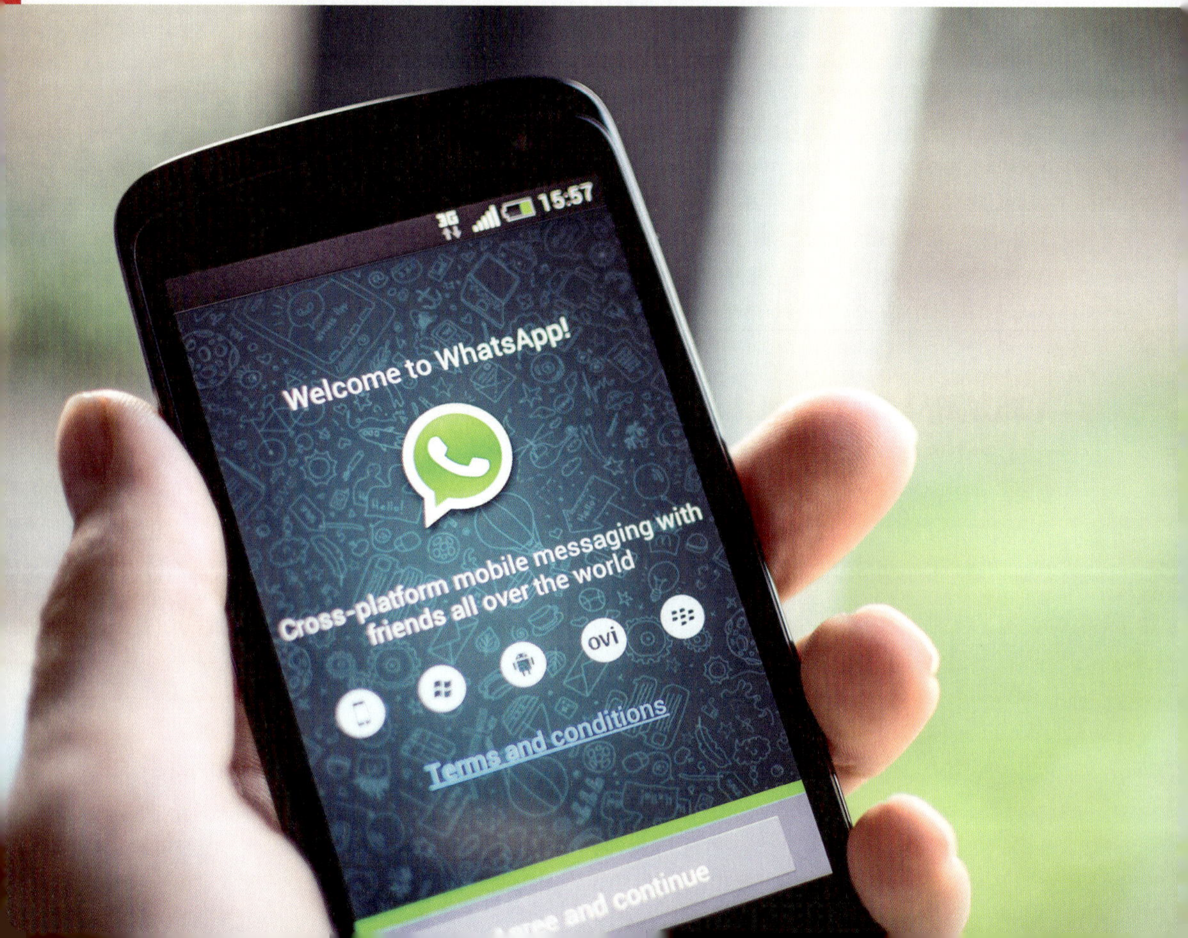

41 percent of teens use messaging apps that automatically delete sent messages. Internet watchdog agency Common Sense Media says there are many reasons why teens have flocked to these apps. They offer unlimited texting and do not deplete the texting limits on many users' cell phone plans. Because each app offers something different, teens enjoy the variety of connections. Many teens also enjoy using apps that are independent of those used by their parents and allow them to be both spontaneous and anonymous.

The Pew survey did not find that text messaging entirely took the place of phone calls for most people. The people who texted more also had the highest rates of phone calls. However, the rate of phone calling is slipping. Twenty-six percent of all teens said they talk daily with friends on their cell phone, down from 38 percent in 2009. Researchers have found that the amount of texting that teens and young adults do appears to correlate with the size of their friend networks. The more friendships teens feel they have to maintain, the more texts they have to initiate and respond to.

Smartphones Have Replaced Older Technology

One of the most important phenomena in the United States in the past few years has been the steep rise in the use of smartphones. These handheld devices have an advanced mobile operating system that acts like a computer. They can connect to the Internet; contain numerous apps; and replace MP3 players, e-readers, and at times even laptop computers. The Pew Research Center reported in 2011 that only 35 percent of Americans owned a smartphone. They were clunky and expensive, adding the cost of additional data plans to monthly mobile phone bills. It did not take long for Americans to realize that easy and convenient access to the Internet was essential. Just four years later, 68 percent of Americans owned a smartphone. Each year the processing speed and power increases and the batteries last longer. Even though screens are getting larger, the devices themselves are getting lighter and slimmer.

Smartphone statistics contrast sharply with ownership of other devices. For instance, from 2011 to 2015, the percentage of adults in the U.S. who owned portable gaming devices such as the Nintendo 3DS declined from 18 percent to 14 percent. The percentage of adults who owned MP3 players such as iPods declined from 44 percent to 40 percent. Even ownership of desktop and laptop computers declined, from a high of 80 percent in 2012 to 73 percent in 2015. From cameras to calculators, smartphones are replacing dozens of older technologies with a device that fits in a pocket.

Teens have found that Internet-connected mobile devices are ideal for their active lifestyles. In 2015 the Pew Research Center reported that 73 percent of teens used a smartphone. African American teens are the most likely of any group of teens to use a smartphone—85 percent, compared with 71 percent of white and Latino teens. According to Pew researcher Amanda Lenhart, "92% of teens report going online daily—including 24% who say they go online 'almost constantly.'"[5] A 2016 media use survey by Common Sense Media found that teens spend almost nine hours each day using their smartphones. Many device users expressed concern about the time they spend on their smartphones. Half of the parents in the survey and one-third of teens said that they were trying to cut down on the amount of time they spend on their devices.

> **"92% of teens report going online daily—including 24% who say they go online 'almost constantly.'"[5]**
>
> —Amanda Lenhart is a researcher at the Pew Research Center.

The "App Generation"

Mobile devices support their users in almost all aspects of life. Most smartphone and tablet owners use apps on their devices to access e-mail, conduct Internet searches, and catch up with the news. In fact, a 2015 Yahoo! analysis found that 90 percent of mobile device users' time is spent on apps. Almost all teens and young adults use apps to access social media sites. Most watch videos and listen to music or podcasts. Many play games. Harvard psychologist Howard Gardner, who researched the impact of mobile devices on teens and young adults, calls these digital natives the "App Generation." He found that "teens and young adults have come to think of the world as an ensemble of apps, to see their lives as a string of ordered apps."[6]

Mobile device users spend large amounts of time using apps to connect with friends and family. The popularity of social media is reflected in a list of most-used apps compiled by online tech news outlet Quartz. The site ranked Facebook as the most popular app used in the United States in 2015, at 125.7 million individual accounts. Seventy-one percent of smartphone users, including teens, accessed the mobile Facebook app daily. A 2015 Pew survey reported that many teens had large networks of Facebook friends. The typical teen had 145 friends. After Facebook, Quartz listed other popular apps regularly used by mobile devices users. The video-sharing site YouTube was listed as the second-most popular, with 98.9 million users. Google apps Search, Play, Maps, and Gmail rounded out the list of most widely used mobile device apps.

Surveys show that Instagram has become one of the most popular apps for teens and young adults. The photo-sharing application calls itself "a fun and quirky way to share your life with

The popular app Instagram (pictured) enables users to take photos with a mobile device and share them with selected followers. More than half of teens use Instagram, and the number of adult users is growing steadily.

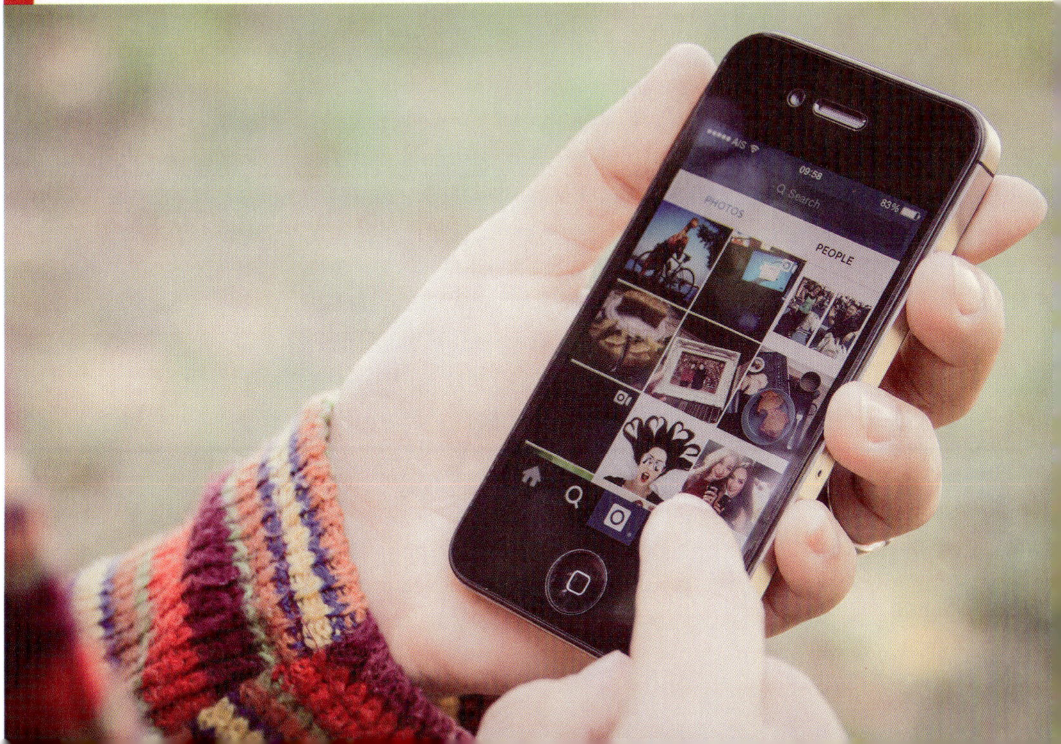

Smartphone Users May Be Learning New Skills at the Expense of Forgetting Old Skills

Because smartphones are able to do so many tasks for users, experts worry that people may be growing up without the skills older generations took for granted. For example, many people rely on their contacts list for telephone numbers instead of remembering them. While it is relatively easy to retrieve a contacts list if a mobile phone is lost or stolen, knowing some important phone numbers might be necessary in an emergency.

Another missing skill is that of reading maps. Map apps such as Google Maps or Maps for iOS give step-by-step directions for finding a new place. However, educators say that many children are not learning how to use physical maps to plot a location, use legends, or figure out scale. Map skills could be crucial if a driver's phone battery dies in an unfamiliar place. Practicing with physical maps occasionally will keep those skills alive.

Because of the ease of texting and e-mailing to contact others, some people avoid making phone calls. According to social psychologist Heidi Grant Halvorson, "If your dominant form of communication with people hasn't been the phone, then you're going to naturally be more anxious using that form of communication." Talking to people on the phone is an essential career skill, she warns young adults new to the business world. She advises that phone call phobics create a script, learn to focus on the phone call recipient, and practice as often as possible.

Quoted in Rachel Sugar, "Why Millennials Are Scared of Talking on the Phone—and How to Get Over It," Business Insider, May 9, 2015. www.businessinsider.com.

friends."[7] After using their mobile device to shoot photos, users can apply different filters to customize them and then leave them public by default or share them with selected followers. Video is available as well. Pew reports that 52 percent of teens use Instagram, with older girls being the heaviest users and having the most followers. Among older adult populations, Instagram is gaining in popularity. Twenty-six percent of adults had accounts in 2014, up from only 13 percent in 2012.

Two applications that are gaining in popularity, particularly among more affluent teen users, are Snapchat and Twitter. Users who receive a photo taken with Snapchat can only view it for a short time, from one to ten seconds. Then it is deleted. When Snapchat first debuted, social media experts were concerned that it would be used for sexting or bullying, since the incriminating evidence would disappear. However, a 2014 University of Washington survey found that most people used the app for fun rather than sending sensitive or inappropriate pictures or information. Twitter is a microblogging site used for posting short messages. They can be public or private, depending on the users' settings.

Mobile device owners who use social media and microblogging apps share details about their personal lives with their networks of family and friends. The media news organization Social Times reported in 2014 that 43 percent of social media users shared photos, which led the list of most-shared items. Opinions, status updates, and links to articles and videos followed at 26 percent each. When US users shared videos, they were most likely to be news clips. In contrast, users in India shared film trailers, and Indonesians shared fashion content. Worldwide, the number one event that was most frequently shared using social media was a relationship status change such as getting engaged or married.

> **"Teens and young adults have come to think of the world as an ensemble of apps, to see their lives as a string of ordered apps."[6]**
>
> —Howard Gardner is a Harvard University psychologist.

Playing games using apps has become a popular leisure activity for mobile device users. Tech industry website CNET reported in 2015 that more children and teens played games on mobile devices than on computers or video game consoles. Sixty-three percent of young gamers played on small screens, compared to 45 percent who used a desktop or laptop computer and 60 percent who played on game consoles. Children and teens also spent more time playing games on mobile devices than in previous years, with an average of six hours each week. Game developers are responding to the improved graphics capability in smartphones. Consumers can buy game controllers with a cradle on the top that turns a smartphone into a gaming console. Other controllers connect to tablets with Bluetooth technology. Gaming giants such as Sony, Microsoft, and Nintendo are turning their attention to the smartphone market with mobile versions of their most popular games.

It is not just teens who have succumbed to the appeal of mobile devices loaded with apps. Babies, toddlers, and preschoolers are spending an increasing amount of time interacting with small screens. A 2016 study published in the journal *Pediatrics* found that 20 percent of one-year-olds owned their own tablet computer. That rate jumped to 75 percent for four-year-olds. Children are learning to use mobile devices at a young age. The survey showed that 28 percent of two-year-olds could navigate a mobile device with no help. The survey found that tablets were displacing television as the major source of media consumption among preschool children.

Mobile Devices Have Become Lifelines

Besides being used to post opinions and images or to engage with a host of entertainments, mobile devices serve as lifelines that connect users to a wide variety of services and information. For instance, a 2015 Pew Technology Device Ownership report showed that 62 percent of smartphone owners used their device to look up information about a health condition. Sixty-seven percent of Americans used mobile banking, 43 percent looked up job information, and 43 percent searched for jobs. Other uses included accessing public transportation information and taking a class. Two-thirds of smartphone users have relied on their devices for directions. More than 70 percent of mobile phone owners used them to track breaking news.

Mobile devices have become even more important to the 10 percent of American smartphone owners who do not have any other form of high-speed Internet access at home beyond their device's data plan. According to the Pew Research Center, these users cannot afford a wired or wireless Internet subscription. Fifteen percent of mobile device users say they have limited ways of getting online other than their smartphone. Many of these

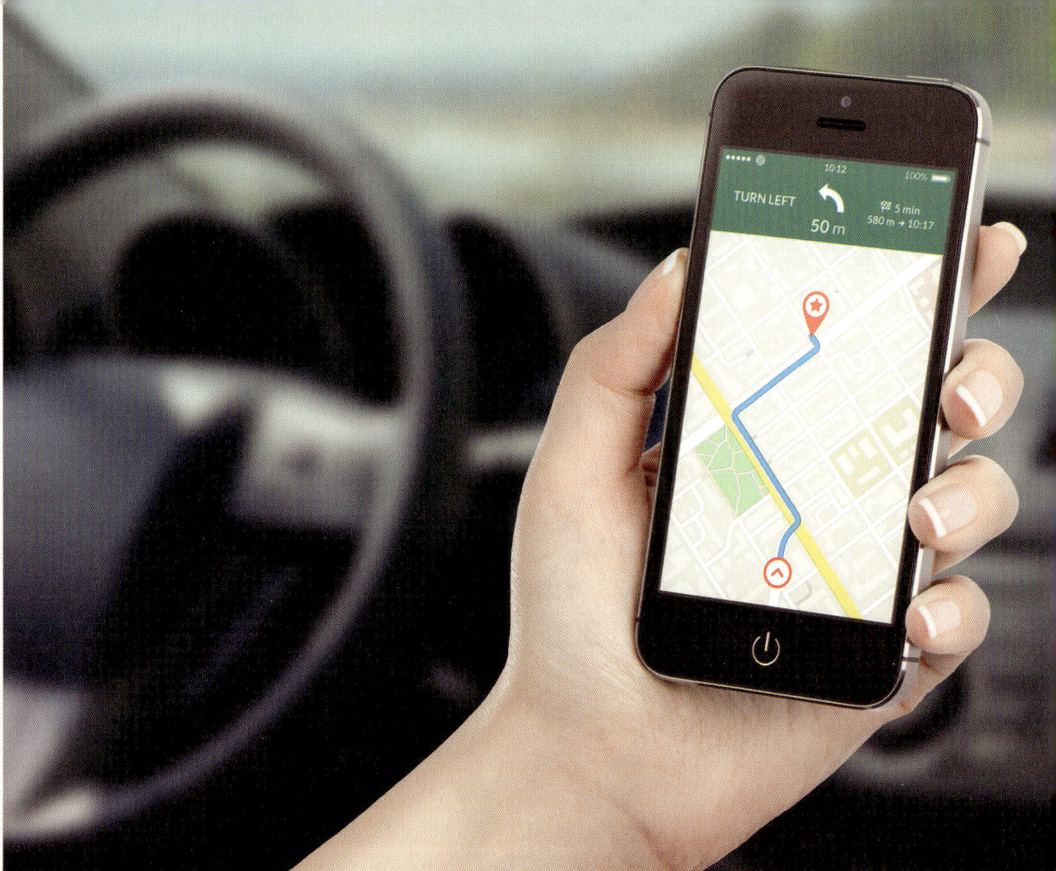

Besides providing entertainment, mobile devices serve as lifelines to connect users to a variety of information and services, such as supplying directions to a destination. These capabilities are particularly useful to the 10 percent of smartphone owners who have no Internet service beyond their device's data plan.

"smartphone-dependent" Americans are those with a low income and low level of education. Smartphone-dependent individuals are less likely to own a home computer, have a bank account, or own their home. Their mobile devices are their primary connection to the online world.

The Future of Mobile Devices

Mobile device developers continue to look for ways to make the devices faster, more powerful, safer, and more useful. For instance, technology that connects smartphones to eyeglasses and wristwatches is being incorporated into other wearable items. Bike helmets that connect to navigation apps, sports bras that track heart rate, and running shoes that measure stride are all on

Global Positioning Systems Can Be Both Friend and Foe

Most mobile phone users do not question the value of the Global Positioning System–based tracking systems embedded in their devices. This handy feature has a lot of advantages. For instance, it can help mobile phone owners find a lost or stolen phone. As long as the phone is charged and turned on, it can continue to broadcast its signal so it can be located. In addition, many mobile phone users enjoy location-based social networking. Some apps provide information about friends who might be nearby, so they can find each other and meet up. Location-based games need players to be near each other to play, encouraging players to get away from their computers and socialize. And more than half of mobile phone users take advantage of navigation features to provide turn-by-turn directions.

However, there is a downside to phone tracking devices. Businesses can take advantage of location-based technology to flood nearby users with advertisements. They can track users to build a profile of users' real-world habits to sell to other advertisers. Strangers may be able to gain access into users' location-based social networking programs. Thieves can follow potential targets to break into their homes while the homeowners are away, broadcasting their whereabouts using location-based apps such as Foursquare or Facebook. Experts advise mobile device users to be prudent with their privacy settings so that only close friends and family can find them.

the horizon. Modular smartphones will allow consumers to build a device that meets their needs. This will reduce waste by allowing users to just replace a malfunctioning component rather than buying a new device. Smartphone materials will become more flexible. Users will be able to fold up their phone into a wallet-sized box or bend it around their wrist as a wristband. Developers predict that virtual reality headsets will use smartphones as their processors and display units. Augmented reality using smartphones will also be common. Using this technology, users can point their device at a movie poster and pull up trailers, games, discount coupons, websites, and reviews. Focusing a device on a foreign language text can immediately pull up a translation. Some technology experts envisage a future in which mobile devices will be part of everything people do.

Mobile technology has become an integral part of life around the globe. Americans are abandoning wired telephones and desktop computers in favor of the ease and portability of smartphones. They are developing and using mobile applications for daily life, entertainment, and connection. Teens are becoming almost constantly connected to the Internet, sending and receiving texts and photos at lightning rates. Mobile devices are changing lives in developing countries as Asians, Africans, and South Americans connect to business, agricultural, and educational resources. Even technology experts are incredulous at how fast the planet has embraced such a close relationship with mobile devices.

2 CHAPTER Do Mobile Phones Impair Users' Physical Health?

In 2009 Italian businessman Innocenzo Marcolini applied for financial compensation from the Italian Workers' Compensation Authority. He had developed a tumor on the left side of his head after holding his mobile phone there for up to six hours a day for twelve years. Though the tumor was benign, the surgery to remove it paralyzed his face, leaving him unable to work. The authority rejected his application, saying there was no proof his illness was caused by his phone. Marcolini appealed to the Italian courts, which reversed the denial of the claim. The Italian Supreme Court was even bold enough to rule that there was a causal link between the use of mobile phones and tumors. This case exemplifies one of the gravest concerns some cell phone users have about their devices—whether long-term use can lead to cancer. However, this concern is only one of the health issues debated over phone use.

Electromagnetic Radiation and Cancer

Whether mobile phones cause cancer has been subject to controversy since the 1990s. The concern arises from the radiation they emit. Mobile devices are a source of electromagnetic radiation (EMR). EMR is all around. Radio waves, microwave ovens, sunlight, and X-rays are all examples of common sources of EMR in people's daily lives. EMR comes in two types. Ionizing radiation causes changes to atoms. Sources of this kind of radiation include the type of X-rays used to diagnose disease, radiation caused by splitting atoms for nuclear weapons, and the gamma rays that come from outer space. Exposure to ionizing radiation can cause damage to living cells, which leads to cancer and other diseases. Nonionizing radiation, such as the type that heats food in a microwave oven or carries sound to a radio, is the type of EMR emitted by mobile devices.

Also called radio-frequency radiation, nonionizing radiation can also have harmful effects. This type of radiation can heat tissue rapidly, especially when EMR-emitting devices are placed next to the skin. Some users have an uncomfortable feeling when they place a cell phone to their ear. They wonder if the source of EMR radiation is too close to the soft tissue of the brain. The long-term effect of this radiation on such tissues is at the center of people's concerns, and it remains the subject of much research as well as debate.

Looking for a Causal Link

Many scientists, such as those called to testify against Marcolini, do not believe that studies so far show a definitive link between mobile phones and cancerous tumors in the head. They point to several European research studies that have monitored users over more than a decade. One of these, the Interphone study, began in 2000 and followed users in thirteen countries. Researchers collected data for ten years, analyzing the time people spent using mobile devices and the incidence of brain tumors. No relationship between cell phone use and brain tumors was found. The researchers noted, however, that ten years of exposure to EMR may not be enough time for tumors to form.

> **"There is no evidence to support the belief that low-level electromagnetic field exposure from electronics, mobile phones and wireless networks are detrimental to health, including the risk of cancer."[8]**
>
> —Dr. Jan Alexander is assistant director general at the Norwegian Institute of Public Health.

In another study published in 2011, researchers in Denmark compared cell phone data with a national cancer registry over a twenty-year period. They also found no association between the use of cell phones and incidents of tumors or cancer. A 2012 study by the Norwegian Institute of Public Health investigated the health risks of exposure to the EMR emitted by mobile phones, cordless landline phones, and cordless phone base stations. Likewise, this study did not find any health risks associated with these devices. Dr. Jan Alexander, lead researcher, concluded, "There is no evidence to support the belief that low-level electromagnetic field exposure

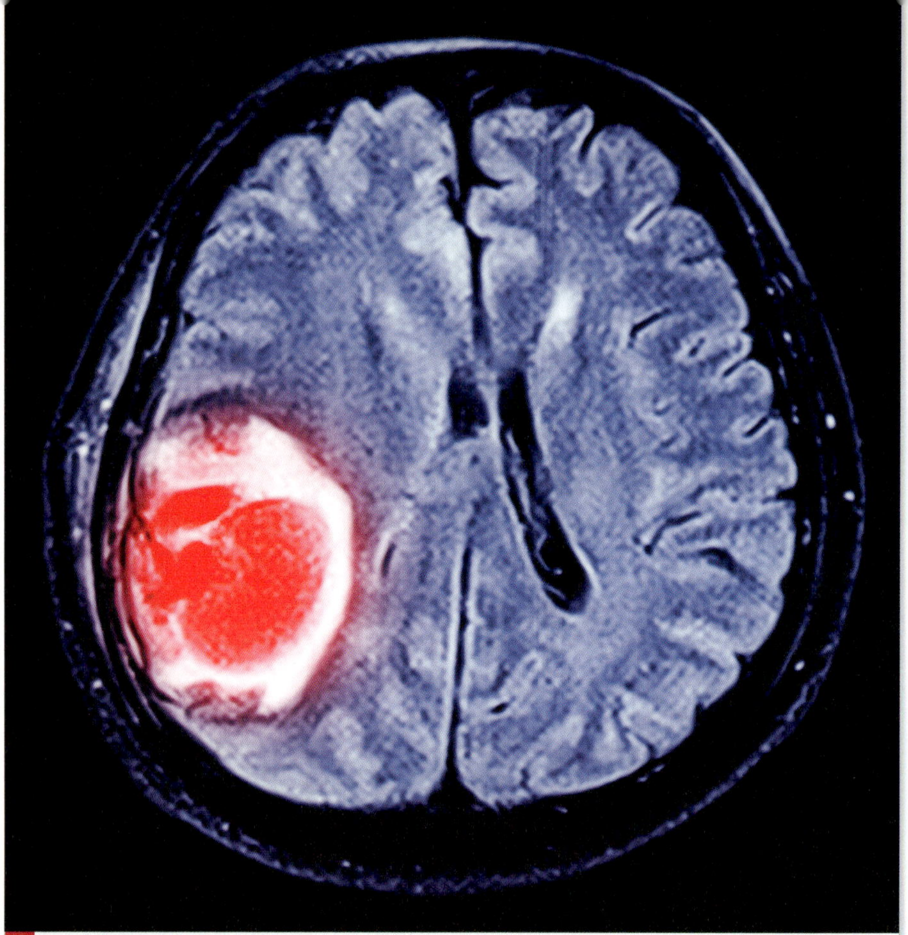

This MRI photo of a human brain shows a tumor, which is depicted in red. Despite claims that mobile phone use causes cancer, many studies have found no definitive link between the two. However, since other studies contradict these, the issue is still hotly debated.

from electronics, mobile phones and wireless networks are detrimental to health, including the risk of cancer."[8]

Several US organizations have weighed in on this issue. The American Cancer Society found no increase in the brain cancer rate between 1987 and 2005, despite a dramatic increase in mobile phone usage during that time. It concludes that currently the evidence is not strong enough to say that cell phones contribute to cancer. The National Institute of Environmental Health Sciences also found no link between mobile technology and cancer. The Centers for Disease Control and Prevention states that current research does not support a significant association between cancer and mobile devices.

Calling Some Studies into Question and Putting Forth New Evidence

Despite these assessments, many scientists have looked at the available research and have come to the opposite conclusion. They believe that much previous research has been flawed or that particular details have been intentionally overlooked. For instance, the scientists point out that the Danish study only looked at whether a citizen had a mobile subscription or not, instead of investigating how the study participants used the phones. They also noted that the Interphone study was funded by a consortium of mobile phone manufacturers, which might have biased the study.

The scientists also point to data in the Interphone study showing that mobile device users of more than ten years were 40 percent more likely to develop a certain kind of malignant brain tumor called a glioma. In another example of overlooked data, Israeli scientists pulled out data from the Interphone study and found that Israeli heavy phone users had a 58 percent higher risk of tumors in the parotid gland. This gland is located right below the ear and produces saliva. Ronald Herberman, director of the University of Pittsburgh Cancer Institute, says of these early efforts, "Most studies claiming that there is no link between cell phones and brain tumors are outdated, had methodological concerns, and did not include sufficient numbers of long term users."[9]

> **"Most studies claiming that there is no link between cell phones and brain tumors are outdated, had methodological concerns, and did not include sufficient numbers of long term users."[9]**
>
> —Ronald Herberman is director of the University of Pittsburgh Cancer Institute.

Scientists who believe in a link between mobile phones and cancer pull evidence from several recent studies. One Swedish study published in 2014 matched 1,380 patients with malignant brain tumors to people without such tumors and compared their wireless phone use. The study included both cordless landline phones and cell phones because both types emit EMR. The results showed that those who used the wireless devices for more

VIEWPOINT

Mobile Devices Can Be Beneficial for Young Children

A 2014 survey found that 38 percent of babies under two years old use tablets or smartphones. Physicians Jenny Radesky, Jayna Schumacher, and Barry Zuckerman from the Division of Developmental Behavior Pediatrics at Boston Medical Center think there are some benefits to allowing the use of digital devices by small children.

> Promising research suggests that interactive media such as learn-to-read apps and electronic books (e-books) may increase early literacy skills by providing practice with letters, phonics, and word recognition. E-books can be useful in promoting vocabulary development and reading comprehension and could be more engaging for young children via digital scaffolds (e.g., oral narration, synchronous text highlighting, and embedded sound effects, animations, or games). Mobile and interactive media have great potential to promote learning through joint engagement between caregivers and children, by demonstrating ideas for parent-child activities, or by modeling teaching strategies (e.g., dialogic reading, phonetic, or sound blending skills) with which low-literacy parents may not be familiar.

Jenny Radesky et al., "Mobile and Interactive Media Use by Young Children: The Good, the Bad, and the Unknown," *Pedatrics*, January 2015.

than twenty-five years were three times more likely to develop a glioma. Most of the patients who developed gliomas began their wireless device use in their teens. It was this research study that influenced the Italian judges to rule in Marcolini's favor; a similar French study the previous year found that mobile device users with more than nine hundred hours of lifetime use had three times the incidence of gliomas.

A Need for More Research

Because of the conflicting research conclusions, both American and European agencies and organizations are currently conducting more studies on the safety of mobile devices. The International

Cohort Study on Mobile Phone Users is monitoring three hundred thousand adult cell phone users in Europe for up to thirty years. Another study called MOBI-KIDS is taking a closer look at children. This international project is looking at the impact of EMR on the risk of brain cancer from exposure of radio-frequency fields throughout childhood and adolescence. Data from one thousand young people aged ten to twenty-four years from sixteen countries is being collected by the Centre for Research in Environmental Epidemiology, based in Spain. The researchers are comparing

VIEWPOINT

Mobile Devices Have Detrimental Effects on Young Children

Some childhood educators do not think that young children should spend time on digital devices. Experts from the Campaign for a Commercial-Free Childhood, Alliance for Childhood, and Teachers Resisting Unhealthy Children's Entertainment believe that too much screen time for infants and toddlers can impact their healthy development.

> Studies show that the more time infants, toddlers, and preschoolers spend with screens, the less time they spend engaged in two activities essential to healthy development and learning. Screen-time takes children away from hands-on creative play—the kind of give-and-take activities that children generate and control and that are specific to their interests and abilities. Newer technologies may also interfere with parent-child conversations. The so-called interactive electronic books—in which screen images respond to touch with sound effects or words or simple movements—are less likely to induce the kind of adult-child interactions that promote literacy than traditional books do.

Campaign for a Commercial-Free Childhood, Alliance for Childhood, and Teachers Resisting Unhealthy Children's Entertainment, "Facing the Screen Dilemma: Young Children, Technology and Early Education," October 2012. www.commercialfreechildhood.org.

those with brain tumors to those who are healthy in hopes of finding or dismissing a link between cell phone use and cancer.

In the meantime, American communities and some European countries are warning their citizens about the potential dangers associated with mobile device use. For instance, in 2015 the cities of Berkeley and San Francisco, both in California, passed an ordinance requiring cell phone retailers to advise customers about the dangers of carrying cell phones close to their bodies. Several US lawmakers have sponsored legislation in Congress asking the Federal Communications Commission to revise its safety limits for mobile device radiation and require health warning labels on all new mobile devices. Internationally, the World Health Organization (WHO) has classified mobile phones as a possible carcinogen. In 2015 a group of 190 scientists from thirty-nine nations asked the United Nations and WHO to strengthen the exposure guidelines for EMR to better protect consumers from potential health risks.

Until the research provides conclusive evidence that mobile devices do not cause cancer, experts recommend that device users follow prudent guidelines. They suggest that users text or use speakerphones or hands-free devices whenever possible. If they need to hold the phone near their ear, they should follow their cell phone manufacturers' guidelines, which caution users to keep phones at least 1 inch (2.5 cm) away from contact with skin and switch ears frequently.

Impact on Physical Fitness

While the potential impact of mobile devices on cancer rates is a cause for concern, many health care professionals are also concerned about these devices' impact on the physical fitness of their users. It has been well known for decades that an inactive lifestyle can have a negative effect on health. People who have sedentary lifestyles are at risk for obesity, cardiovascular problems, diabetes, and other diseases. Many health care professionals question whether mobile devices lead to a sedentary lifestyle or whether the devices can be a valuable aid to encourage physical fitness.

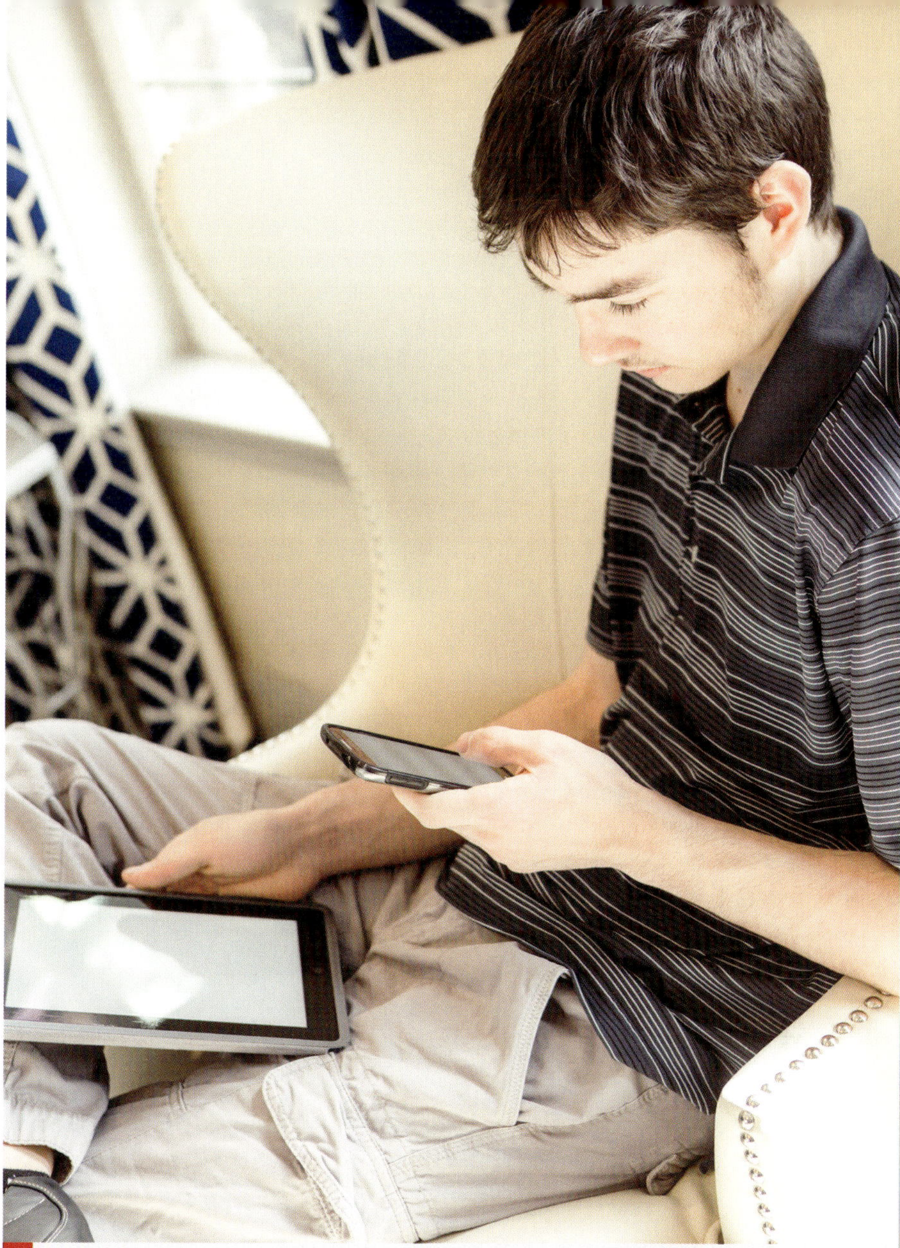

Some research has shown that heavy users of mobile devices are less physically active than less frequent users. However, fitness apps and wearable fitness technologies may play a part in reversing this trend.

Some researchers claim that the increasing use of mobile devices among teens and young adults has led to an increase in inactivity. One 2013 study of students at a midwestern university examined the relationship between cell phone use and physical pursuits. The researchers hypothesized that the more students used their phones, the lower their physical activity levels. That is indeed what they found. On average, the students used their phones for five hours each day, primarily for leisure activities such as texting, updating social media, surfing the Internet, and playing games. Students who used their phones the least reported that they participated in more physical activities than those who used their phones the most.

On the other hand, companies behind the recent development of fitness apps and wearable fitness technologies claim that smartphone apps can reverse the trends toward inactivity. These apps connect to gadgets that strap on to wrists or clip on to belt loops. The devices count steps, track heart rate, measure calories burned, and collect data that can be sent to physicians and health coaches. They also connect users to communities that provide motivation. "I started wearing UP in September, and that's when I started working out and being healthy,"[10] one customer says about his experience using the Jawbone technology company's fitness wristband. Another wearable fitness tracker maker, Fitbit, claims on its website that 78 percent of Fitbit users say their activity level has increased since using their devices. A 2015 study titled "Wearable Fitness Trackers Inspire More Active Behavior" found promising results. Eighty-five percent of users reported they increased the distance they ran or walked, and 86 percent increased the overall amount of physical activity each week. However, the study was funded by the Consumer Technology Association, an organization of companies that make fitness gadgets and apps, which has prompted accusations that the report was biased.

Most fitness experts say that whether wearable fitness technologies and apps can increase physical activity depends on factors such as user support and motivation and the devices' ease of use and reliability. A 2015 study conducted by the University of Pennsylvania School of Medicine found that one-third of people using fitness trackers stop using them after six months, and one half do so after a year. Some reasons for abandoning the devices include losing them, technical problems with the device or website, and concern about the privacy of the data collected. Many health professionals and app developers are optimistic, however, that they can overcome these problems and produce solutions that will get mobile device users off the couch and into the gym.

Impact on Sleep

While mobile device users debate whether their devices impact their physical fitness, many agree that there is one area where their devices are having a negative impact. That is on their sleep. Many people use their devices before going to sleep to read, listen to music, watch videos, and chat with family and friends. The impact of devices on sleep is particularly severe for young users. A 2012 Time/Qualcomm survey found that a quarter of respondents aged eighteen to twenty-four agreed with the statement "I don't sleep as well as I used to because I am connected to technology all the time."[11]

Some researchers claim that mobile devices can seriously impair sleep. A 2014 Penn State University study compared adults who read on an iPad before sleep each night for a week

Teen girls check their smartphones before going to sleep. Researchers warn that the negative effects mobile devices have on sleep may lead to severe long-term health problems.

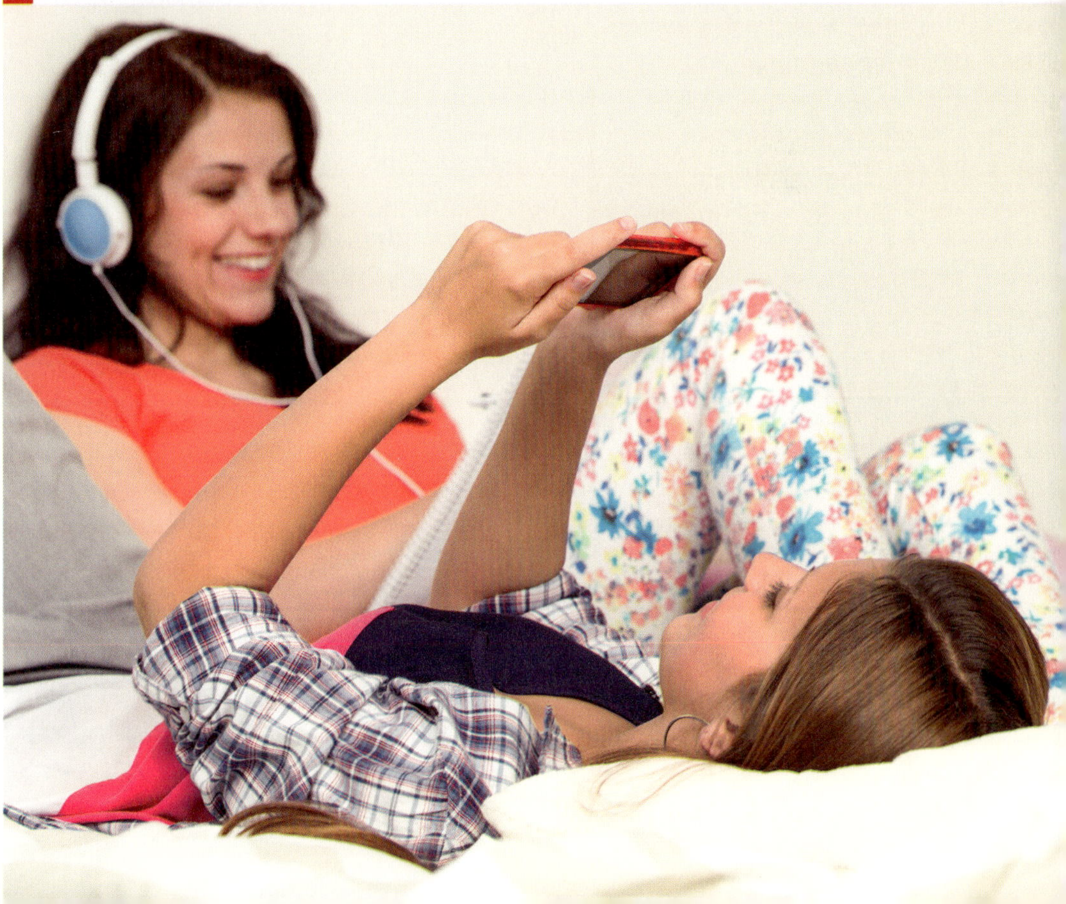

with those who read using a print book. Digital devices such as smartphones, tablets, and light-emitting diode (LED) computer monitors emit blue light. Blue light can have a negative effect on people's melatonin levels. This hormone typically increases in the evening and helps people fall asleep. Researchers found that the iPad readers had reduced levels of melatonin and took longer to fall asleep. They also spent less time in rapid-eye-movement sleep, the kind of sleep that helps restore cells. They reported being sleepier and less alert the following morning.

The researchers warned that sleep loss due to electronic devices could lead to long-term health problems. Chronic suppression of melatonin has been linked to increased risk of breast, prostate, and colorectal cancers. Because hormones involved with appetite suppression are active during sleep, lack of sleep has been associated with diabetes and obesity. Dr. Charles Czeisler, director of the Division of Sleep Medicine at Harvard Medical School, says, "We introduce these devices that have medical and biological effects without requiring any health studies on their impact. . . . They don't have to go through any evaluation like a drug would, for safety and efficacy. I think it's time to rethink that."[12]

"We introduce these devices that have medical and biological effects without requiring any health studies on their impact. . . . They don't have to go through any evaluation like a drug would, for safety and efficacy."[12]

—Charles Czeisler is director of the Division of Sleep Medicine at Harvard Medical School.

A 2014 study of Australian teens also found negative effects of mobile device use before sleep. The Woolcock Institute of Medical Research in Australia surveyed 11,500 eleven- to seventeen-year-olds. In addition to the harmful impact of reduced melatonin on maintaining circadian rhythms, researchers found that the interactivity of mobile devices kept users alert for longer times. They hypothesize that midnight checking of social media fails to create an association between bed and sleep. Study leader Dr. Nathaniel Marshall proposed that the concept of FOMO—fear of missing out—keeps teens on favorite Internet sites longer than is healthy. He explains, "We suspect that many of these overtired kids are driven to stay up late texting, chatting, and gaming with mates on their phone, computer, or tablet just so they're in the loop with what's going on."[13]

While there is no technological remedy for FOMO, there may be solutions to the blue light issue. Application developers have created software that can be installed on laptops that calibrates the devices' color displays to the time of day. At sunset, the program changes the blue light to warmer colors to reduce any impact on melatonin. Filters are also available that can be put on top of tablet and cell phone screens to reduce the effect of blue light.

Research is still ongoing as to whether mobile devices have an impact on physical health. It may take decades to determine what, if any, effects cell phones have on cancer, obesity, or sleep. Future electronic engineers may design mobile devices that are safe and promote a healthy lifestyle. Device users who are educated on the risks of new technology will be able to make better decisions regarding their health.

Chapter 3 Are Mobile Devices a Dangerous Distraction?

Anyone walking or driving along the Avenues section of Salt Lake City, Utah, in June 2013 would have been forgiven for doing a double take and staring at the driver of a silver 2010 Subaru Outback. The University of Utah volunteer's head was covered with an electroencephalograph cap, and additional electrodes were placed around each eye. A band around her head held a GoPro camera. Another head-mounted device held an LED light in her peripheral vision. Four LifeCam USB cameras were arranged around the front cabin to capture the driver's facial expressions. Wires snaked out of the brake and gas pedals as well as the steering wheel. A passenger in the backseat wielded a laptop and more equipment. The student was participating in an experiment conducted by Dr. David Strayer and his team at the Applied Cognition Lab at the University of Utah. The research was sponsored by the American Automobile Association (AAA), which was concerned about the proliferation of car "infotainment" systems and their potential to distract drivers.

In recent years more and more states have been addressing the issue of distracted driving caused by the use of mobile devices. Research studies and evidence from law enforcement agencies in the past decade convinced many state legislatures to pass laws against texting via handheld devices while driving. Drivers responded by switching their mobile device use to hands-free mode. They use headsets with microphones or their car's smartphone-connected audio system. Some transportation experts claim that these new systems have solved the distracted driving problem by keeping drivers' eyes on the road and their hands on the steering wheel. Other experts, such as Strayer and his team, disagree. They set out to show that hands-free mobile device use is just as dangerous as handheld use.

The Subaru's driver was asked to do eight tasks, all while being monitored by high-tech equipment that allowed the team to assess what was going on in her brain and where her eyes tracked. The first task, just driving, created baseline data. Then the driver was asked to drive while listening to the radio, listening to a book on tape, talking with a passenger, talking on a handheld cell phone, talking on a hands-free cell phone, using the car's speech-to-text e-mail system, and completing an auditory math and memorization task. With the exception of using the handheld phone, all tasks allowed the driver to keep both hands on the steering wheel and both eyes on the road.

Strayer uses the term *cognitive workload* to describe the effort required to concentrate on a task such as driving. He was trying to find out whether using the car's hands-free systems was safer than using a handheld device. His experiments measured how much the tasks suppressed brain activity in areas needed for safe driving, increased reaction time, resulted in missed stop signs and other visual cues, and decreased visual scanning of the driving environment. He created a scale of cognitive distraction from a level of one for just driving to a level of five for driving while solving math problems and memorizing lists of words. After analyzing the data from his experiments, he published his findings

A teen talks on the phone while driving. Although many states permit the use of hands-free devices behind the wheel, some studies suggest that the use of such devices is only marginally less distracting to drivers than using handheld ones.

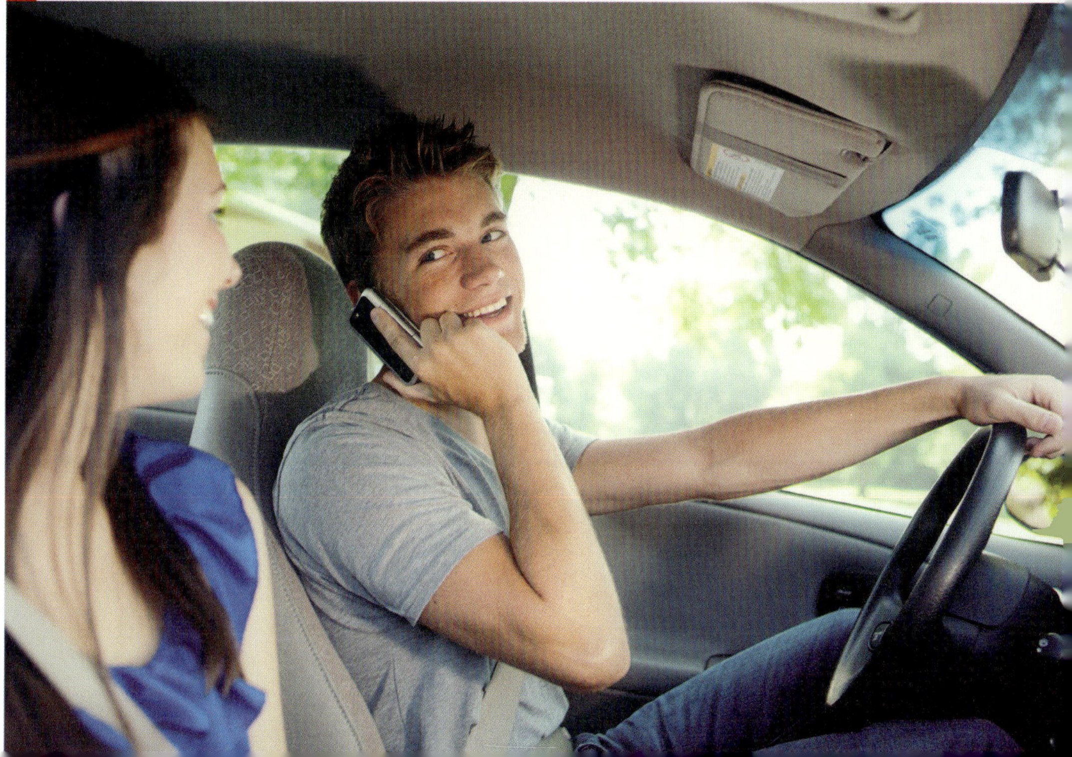

in a report called "Measuring Cognitive Distraction in the Automobile." His results surprised both experts and the general public, who assumed that hands-free tasks were safe. The experiment showed that listening to the radio or book on tape did not suppress brain activity. However, the more complex tasks moved the brain's attention from driving to the tasks. Strayer believes that these experiments proved that operating a car's audio system to access texting, e-mail, and other smartphone apps takes a driver's attention away from the primary task of driving.

Early Research on Distracted Driving

One of the earliest studies on the impact of mobile devices on driving was conducted in 1997 by researchers Donald Redelmeier and Robert Tibshirani. Analyzing 699 drivers with cell phones who had crashed their cars, they found that the risk of driving while talking on phones was four times higher than without the phone—the same risk as with driving impaired by alcohol. A 2001 study supported Redelmeier and Tibshirani's findings. Carnegie Mellon University scientists found that participating in a conversation significantly distracts the brain from processing visual information. They used functional magnetic resonance imaging to measure brain activity while volunteers tried to do two things at once. The participants were given a visual activity—comparing two three-dimensional objects—while listening to sentences read to them. The brain's visual center activity declined by 29 percent, while auditory activity declined by 53 percent. According to Carnegie Mellon psychology professor Marcel Just, "This has direct implications for cell phone use during driving because it answers one of the classic questions about human thinking. We've demonstrated that the human brain has a limited ability to perform two cognitive tasks concurrently under demanding circumstances, such as simultaneously conversing and driving."[14] The

> **"We've demonstrated that the human brain has a limited ability to perform two cognitive tasks concurrently under demanding circumstances, such as simultaneously conversing and driving."[14]**
>
> —Marcel Just is a psychology professor at Carnegie Mellon University.

researchers found that both driving and the conversation suffered when participants tried to do them both at the same time.

Hands-Free Is as Dangerous as Handheld

As Bluetooth technology became popular, researchers turned their attention to comparing handheld device distraction to that of the new hands-free devices. Drivers began using headsets or car technology that allowed them to keep their phones in their pockets or purses in hopes that this would allow them to keep better control of their autos. However, the idea that hands-free was safer was immediately challenged. A 2005 study published in the *Journal of Neuroscience* found that the brain cannot pay attention to both the visual requirements of driving and the auditory task of following a conversation. The study's authors concluded that talking on a hands-free device was as dangerous as talking on a handheld one.

Some researchers think that there is a "bottleneck" in the brain that prevents people from doing two things at the same time. René Marois, an associate professor of psychology, explains:

> While we are driving, we are bombarded with visual information. We might also be talking to passengers or talking on the phone. Our new research offers neurological evidence that the brain cannot effectively do two things at once. People think if they are using a headset with their cell phone while driving they are safe, but they're not because they are still doing two cognitively demanding tasks at once.[15]

Drivers may be looking at the road, but they are not seeing what is there because their brain is engaged in another task.

More recent research appears to support the earlier findings regarding the safety of hands-free devices. A 2015 study by the AAA Foundation for Traffic Safety compared hands-free technologies in ten vehicles. In these cars, drivers were able to access the text messages and e-mails on their mobile devices through the vehicle's audio system. Researchers assessed the potential for distraction

> **"Tasks that take a driver's eyes off the road or hands off the steering wheel are what increase crash risk. Texting, emailing, manual dialing and so forth—not conversation—are what increase the risk of crashes while driving."[17]**
>
> —Dr. Richard Young is a researcher at Wayne State University.

when using the various technologies. Judged on a six-point distraction scale, with six being the most distracting, the technologies' scores ranged from a low of 2.4 for a Chevy system to a high of 4.6 in that of a Mazda. The lower numbers came from technologies that had fewer errors, required less time to use, and were relatively easy to figure out.

One disturbing finding was what the researchers called the residual effect of using the devices. According to the report:

> The data indicate that just because a driver terminates a call or text message does not mean that they are no longer impaired. Indeed, significant residual costs were observed for 27 seconds after the IVIS [In-Vehicle Information System] interaction had terminated. At the 25 MPH speed limit in our study, drivers would have traveled over the length of three football fields during this interval.[16]

Researchers concluded that during that time, drivers could drive through stop signs or not notice pedestrians while they bring their attention back to driving. The researchers believe that using hand-free mobile devices while driving is dangerous.

Car Crash Rates Decreased Despite Increase in Mobile Devices

Not all transportation experts believe that using mobile devices while driving is a safety risk. Some believe that while handheld devices can cause driver distraction, hands-free device use is safe. Instead of measuring distractions in simulated driving labs or experimental driving tasks, Dr. Richard Young from Wayne State University pored over the General Motors OnStar hands-free communication database looking for air bag deployments occurring at

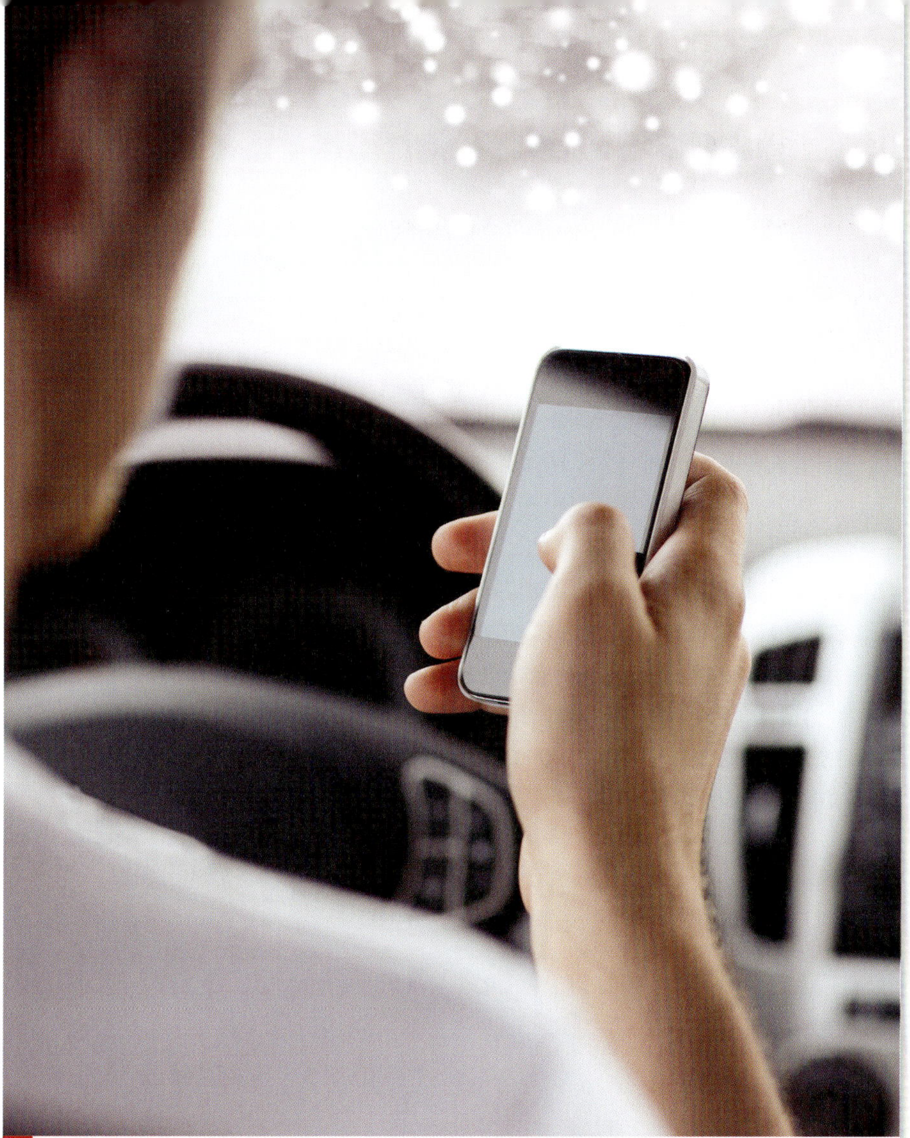

A driver looks at his mobile phone while on the road. Some researchers say that simply having a hands-free conversation by mobile phone is much less dangerous than using the phone to perform any task that takes the driver's attention off the road or hands off the steering wheel.

the same time as a phone call. For their 2009 study, he and his colleagues found only fourteen calls in progress at the time of a crash, at a rate of one crash per 3.3 million calls. "Tasks that take a driver's eyes off the road or hands off the steering wheel are what increase crash risk," says Young. "Texting, emailing, manual dialing and so forth—not conversation—are what increase the risk of crashes while driving."[17]

VIEWPOINT

Laws Banning Cell Phone Use While Driving Recognize the Serious Risks

Many Americans think using a hands-free device to make a phone call is not safe. They would like to see a total ban on making phone calls while driving. One of these is Janet Froetscher, president of the National Safety Council. She explains:

> More than 50 research studies have reported the risks of cellphone use while driving. Talking on a cellphone while driving makes a person four times more likely to be in a crash. This is a much higher risk than most other distracting activities, including eating, drinking, reading billboards, listening to the radio, or talking to other passengers. It's the cellphone conversation that diverts people's attention from the road. The National Safety Council has called for a total ban on cellphone use while driving because more than 100 million people are engaged in this high-risk activity every day. We do not support laws that would permit the use of hands-free devices, because there is no scientific evidence that those devices are any safer for drivers.

Janet Froetscher, "Education, Backed by Law," *Room for Debate* (blog), *New York Times*, July 18, 2009. www.nytimes.com.

Other studies appear to muddy up the distracted driving debate. Distracted driving crash rates do not seem to be increasing with the rise in smartphone ownership. According to the National Highway Traffic Safety Administration (NHTSA), in 2013, 16 percent of police-reported automobile crashes nationwide were coded as distraction-caused crashes, the same rate as in 2009. Nor are teens crashing their cars at high rates because of texting. The NHTSA reports that though a quarter of teens admit to responding to a text message every time they drive, only 10 percent of crashes in that age group are attributed to distracted driving. Another study shows that the most prominent cause of distraction is daydreaming, and the most significant reason for crash fatalities among teens remains lack of seat belt use.

Some researchers use car crash data to support their argument that hands-free mobile device use while driving does not cause crashes. The NHTSA has been collecting statistics about car crash fatalities since 1975. While the rate of mobile device ownership skyrocketed from almost nonexistent in 1975 to more than 90 percent of drivers today, the number of crash fatalities has been cut in half, from twenty per one hundred thousand people to an all-time low of ten per one hundred thousand. A 2013 analysis of teen automobile fatalities by the Insurance Institute for Highway Safety's Highway Loss Data Institute showed that the number of teens dying in car crashes declined 71 percent from 1971 to 2012. The institute's analysis noted that safety features in cars such as air bags and seat belts can account for some but not all of the decrease. Car

VIEWPOINT

Laws Banning Cell Phone Use While Driving Overlook Some Positives

One who disagrees with a ban on phone calls while driving is Katherine Mangu-Ward, a senior editor at *Reason* magazine. She does not believe that talking on the phone is any more dangerous than dozens of other things drivers do while driving, which are not banned by law. She explains:

> **Think of every carpool disaster averted, grocery list amended, or stress-relieving traffic update made possible by the use of cellphones in cars. Think of every kid who got through to his mom, every long-distance relationship maintained, every roadtrip rescued. True, these aren't matters of life and death, but billions of tiny gains in happiness and reductions in stress are too often overlooked in public policy debates.**

Katherine Mangu-Ward, "Let People Dial While Driving," *Room for Debate* (blog), *New York Times*, July 18, 2009. www.nytimes.com.

manufacturers assert that driving has become easier and more automated. They claim that despite the increase in mobile devices, driving has never been safer.

Instead of looking at the overall car crash fatality rate to make an argument about the safety of using hands-free mobile devices while driving, some researchers focus on fatalities due to distracted driving. These statistics further complicate the debate. While all traffic fatalities have gone down in the past two decades, the rates of fatalities from distracted driving appear to be rising. A 2010 study by researchers at the University of North Texas Health Science Center compared the increase in distracted driving fatalities to the increase in cell phone use and texting volume. The researchers obtained Fatality Analysis Reporting System records on all crash fatalities on public roads in the United States from 1999 to 2008. They found that fatalities from distracted driving increased 28 percent after 2005, almost the same rate as the growth of smartphones, text messaging, and the use of mobile devices for e-mailing and accessing social media. Despite the large drop in car crash fatalities in the past four decades, the debate still rages over whether using hand-free mobile devices while driving is safe.

States Pass Cell Phone Restrictions

A debate is also ongoing about what states should do in response to drivers' desires to use mobile devices while driving. As research trickled in about the impact of multitasking on driving, states began passing bans on texting or talking on handheld cell phones while driving. By the beginning of 2016, fourteen states had prohibited all drivers from using handheld cell phones while driving. The laws are primary enforcement laws, which means an officer can stop and cite a driver for using a handheld device without any other traffic offense. Forty-six states banned text messaging for all drivers; thirty-nine of these bans were primary enforcement laws. Thirty-eight states banned all cell phone use for drivers who have a learner's permit or are under age eighteen. Only two states—Montana and Arizona—had no laws against the use of mobile devices while driving (except for school bus drivers).

State laws regulating the use of mobile devices while driving have had little impact on car crashes. The Highway Loss Data Institute, which collects data on insurance claims due to crashes, compared the crash rates of several counties in New Jersey before and after an intense period of enforcement of a handheld cell phone ban from 2009 to 2011. The results were puzzling. While rates of texting and handheld cell phone use went down, the rate of crashes did not—and in some cases they increased. The organization suggested several reasons for these findings. Perhaps some drivers had put their phones on their laps to hide them from law enforcement. Others might have switched to hands-free phone use and were still distracted. Still other drivers might have found other ways to entertain themselves during a tedious drive that were more distracting than using their phones.

A woman waits in her car after being pulled over by a police officer. In fourteen states, laws that prohibit motorists from using handheld cell phones while driving allow officers to stop and cite any driver who does so.

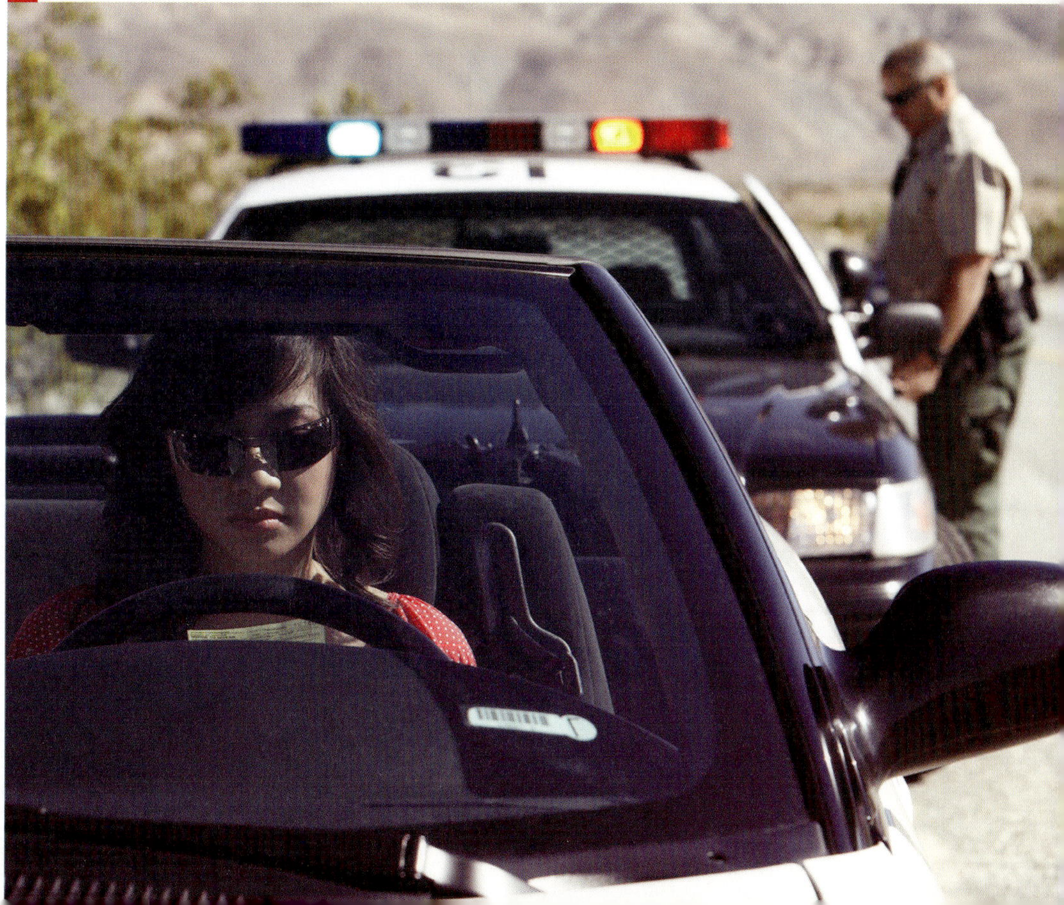

Distracted Driving Solutions

Surveys of mobile device owners show that despite knowing the risks involved, many drivers are not likely to stop using their phones while driving. Public campaigns to reduce distracted driving and increased law enforcement have had only limited and often temporary success. However, automobile engineers, app developers, and device manufacturers are coming up with innovative solutions to reduce distracted driving.

New technologies in cars and smartphones are showing potential in reducing driver distraction. The manufacturer-installed Full Windshield Head-Up Display puts information from drivers' smartphone apps in transparent images on the cars' windshields. Controls are located on the steering wheel. Drivers never have to take their eyes off the road. In addition, some developers have created apps for the Apple iPhone that work in a similar way. When the phone is placed faceup on a car's dashboard, its display projects onto the windshield, giving drivers directions to their destination and information about upcoming hazards.

Perhaps the most promising solution to distracted driving is the self-driving car. Almost every automobile manufacturer is researching autonomous vehicles, working with tech giants such as Google and Tesla. Some experts predict that semiautonomous cars, those with a driver in the car who can take control if necessary, will be common by 2020. Others believe driverless cars are still far off in the future.

However, until drivers can let their vehicles do the driving for them, most experts have clear recommendations about the use of mobile devices while operating the car. Parents need to set clear expectations and enforce rules about their children's use of cell phones while driving. States need to pass and enforce bans against using handheld devices while on the road. And drivers need to take responsibility for preventing distractions while driving.

4 CHAPTER Are People Too Dependent on Mobile Devices?

Mobile device users around the world are beginning to wonder whether they are becoming too dependent on their online connections. Nala Cheng is one example of a teen who is worried about cell phone dependency. She used a youth blogging site to express her concern about the amount of time she and her friends spend on their phones.

> Hi, I'm Nala Cheng, a high school student from Taiwan. For this very first post, I'd like to talk about Disconnect Anxiety. Do you suffer from Disconnect Anxiety? Disconnect anxiety is a feeling of discomfort that occurs when a heavy smartphone user can not access the online world. In the modern society, millions of people are now suffering from it.[18]

In 2015 a Google study found that mobile phone users in developed countries such as Taiwan spent more than three hours each day actively using their devices. College students averaged nine hours per day of device use, while simultaneously studying and socializing. Most of the time was spent using apps such as Instagram, Facebook, Snapchat, Twitter, or Tumblr. Teens and young adults spent a significant amount of time texting, averaging well over one hundred texts each day.

In 2014 the Pew Research Center reported that 93 percent of people surveyed said that they found their mobile devices helpful. For many Americans, their smartphone and its data plan are their only options for online access. They rely on their phone for connecting to work, school, medical care, transportation, and banking. It's the first thing they check in the morning and the last thing they look at before they go to sleep. Increasingly, though, many mobile device users are concerned about the time they spend on their phones. They worry about their constant urge to check their phones, often several times an hour. They feel anxious when

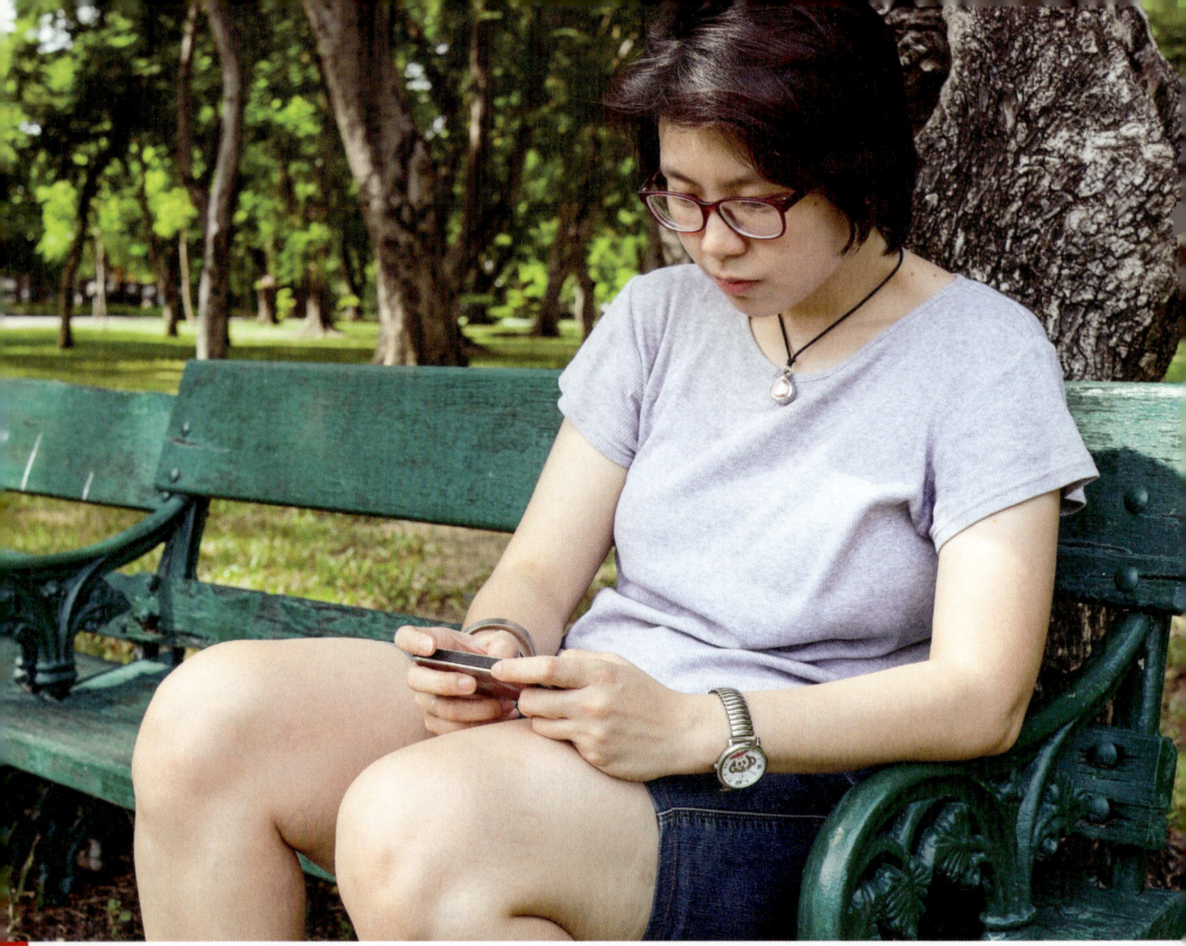

A woman checks messages on a mobile phone. A few experts, but not all, argue that the need to check one's mobile phone constantly is a dependency comparable to opioid addiction.

they are without their phones. One label for this anxiety is nomophobia, or fear of being without one's phone. Some experts go even further. They call the constant phone checking an addiction, claiming that the compulsive behaviors of some cell phone users is similar to opioid users anticipating their next fix.

Mobile Device Dependency and Brain Science

Although it is debatable whether excessive mobile phone use is an addictive behavior, some technology experts have turned to addiction specialists to understand nomophobia. As these experts explain, deep inside everyone's brain is a pleasure center called the nucleus accumbens. When something good happens, the nucleus accumbens is flooded with a substance called dopamine. Dopamine is a neurotransmitter, a chemical produced by neurons in the brain that helps transmit signals between neurons. Neurons that release dopamine work on a reward system, so that when the same pleasurable event happens again, the neurons are ready to respond. People become motivated to keep repeating the event to continue the supply of the neurotransmitter. Drugs and alcohol produce faster, stronger dopamine signals. Even the anticipation of a drug can release dopamine.

Researchers in the past decade have found that some people indulge in compulsive behaviors because they receive similar rewards in their brain's pleasure center. Examples of these behaviors include gambling and playing video games. These behaviors have something else in common that causes the brain to crave them. They both involve uncertainty and unpredictability. The brain loves stimulation, and not knowing the outcome of an event ahead of time sets up anticipation and excitement. According to the researchers, every text message or social media notification lights up the brain's pleasure center.

Because the brain desires both the uncertainty of the outcome and the unpredictability of the reward, Dr. David Greenfield, founder of the Center for Internet and Technology Addiction, calls the smartphone "the world's smallest slot machine."[19] Every time gamblers insert money and push the slot machine's button, they get a squirt of dopamine into their brains' reward system. They do not know whether this play will pay off or how much they will win. If they do hit a jackpot, the reward center gets more dopamine, and the players feel pleasure. They cannot wait to do it again. Scientists call this cycle a feedback loop. "Every time you go on to that smartphone and check something, there is an unpredictability about what you're going to find and how good it's going to be for you,"[20] says Greenfield. Phone users keep checking their phones the way gamblers feed the slot machine. App developers are well aware of this behavior. Internet articles such as "10 Ingredients That Concoct an Addictive Mobile App" or "Hooked: How to Build Habit-Forming Products" show that developers understand and capitalize on the feedback loop.

Mobile Phone Addiction

One person who is convinced that many young people are addicted to their mobile devices is Nashville English teacher Jarred Amato. "There's always a text message to send, there's always a new picture to see, there's always a new Snapchat to send," he says about his ninth graders. "They never get a break. And if you ask them, they really don't like it, but they almost feel powerless to it."[21] In 2015 Amato challenged his students to take a "digital cleanse" and lock up their phones in a classroom cabinet for twenty-four hours. When students arrived in class the next day, Amato noticed a change. "If you looked at this room yesterday, with their phones, the noise level was a lot lower, because they were just consumed with their phone," he said. "Now, look around, see how many conversations you see. Every pocket of the room looking at each other, smiling, laughing, hitting, flirting, all the normal teenage stuff that I think has kind of been forgotten."[22] Students reported that they had dinner with their family instead of in their bedroom, got more sleep, and played outside for the first time in a while.

> **"The words 'addicted' and 'addiction,' 'obsessed' and 'obsessing,' came up again and again in my interviews with more than 200 teenage girls as they talked about their use of the smartphones and consuming media and using social media."[23]**
>
> —Nancy Jo Sales is the author of *American Girls: Social Media and the Secret Lives of Teenagers.*

Author Nancy Jo Sales, in her 2016 book *American Girls: Social Media and the Secret Lives of Teenagers*, found that many of the teens she interviewed considered themselves overly attached to their phones. She says:

> The words "addicted" and "addiction," "obsessed" and "obsessing," came up again and again in my interviews with more than 200 teenage girls as they talked about their use of the smartphones and consuming media and using social media. How else can you characterize an activity that, depending on which study you reference, occupies anywhere from nine to eleven hours of your day?[23]

In 2010 students at the University of Maryland took the lead in a project called the World Unplugged. Similar to the students in Nashville, one thousand college students from twelve universities in ten countries attempted to live without their phones for a day. The study concluded that "students around the world repeatedly used the language of addiction and dependency to speak about their media habits."[24] "Media is my drug; without it I was lost. I am an addict," said a student from the United Kingdom. An American student wrote on her blog, "I was itching, like a crackhead, because I could not use my phone."[25] Other students reported sadness, depression, and distress.

Mobile device app developer Raefer Gabriel blames "the increased use of adaptive, personalized feeds in social media" that give phone users "more incentive to overconsume." Facebook and Twitter provide a constant stream of messages directly relevant to the user. Gabriel says that "when you interrupt the dopamine feedback loop of any sort of pleasure-seeking behavior, you'll see withdrawal symptoms—and people definitely look anxious and moody when you take away their constant smartphone connectivity."[26]

Interfering with Other Tasks

To support the claim that a specific behavior qualifies as an addiction, some experts measure the degree to which it interferes with daily life. A person whose only goal is getting high or winning big at the blackjack table usually exhibits an inability to function well in school, work, social situations, or intimate relationships. Experts are examining mobile device behaviors using similar criteria. They want to know whether mobile devices negatively impact performance on the job, in school, or in relationships.

College professor and researcher Reynol Junco has conducted numerous studies on the effect of engaging in social media while taking notes in class and studying after class. "That absolutely is not a good idea," he said in his 2012 study examining the relationship between multitasking and academic performance. "Do not text or Facebook during class. Do not text or Facebook while you're studying for your classes."[27] Junco's studies showed that students who were checking social media or texting were not able to simultaneously attend to classroom activities or homework assignments. He found that students who multitasked with their phones while in class or doing homework had significantly lower grade point averages.

A teen girl texts during a class. Students who multitask using their mobile phones while doing homework or attending class have lower grade point averages than their peers who do not, according to one study.

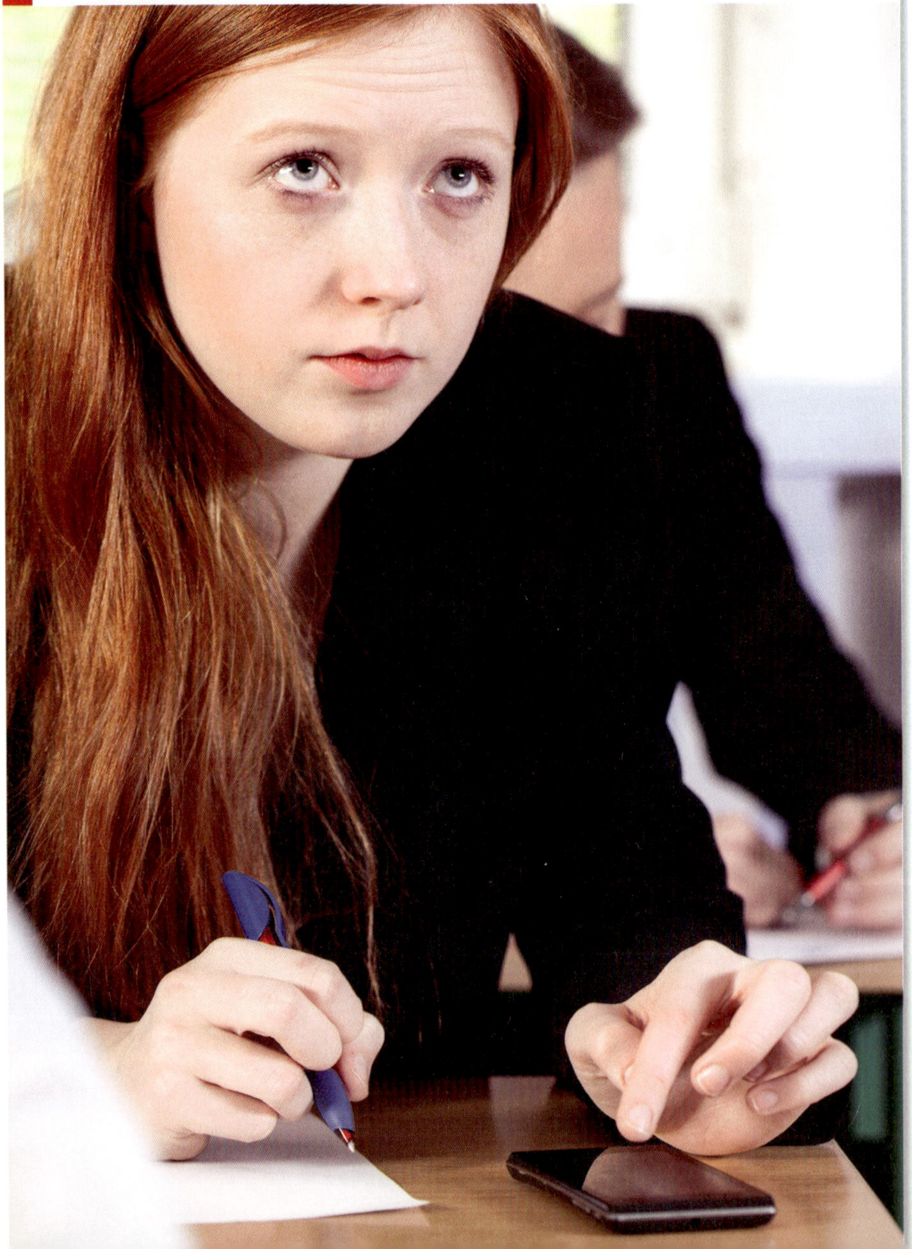

In 2015 researchers at the University of Florida performed an experiment to gauge the extent to which mobile devices distracted workers from completing a task. One group of study participants attempted to complete a computer task while receiving phone calls. Another group received text messages, and the control group received no messages or calls. The students who received calls or texts made many more errors on the task than the control group. The researchers concluded that "cellular notifications, even when one does not view or respond to messages or answer calls, can significantly damage performance on attention-demanding tasks."[28]

Mobile Device Impact on Relationships

Communication skills is another area of daily life in which the negative impact of mobile devices is becoming an issue of concern. Some experts worry that because of constant texting, posting, and instant messaging, people are losing the ability to communicate face-to-face. Massachusetts Institute of Technology professor Sherry Turkle spent five years researching the consequences of communicating by cell phone. She is concerned that teens and young adults are avoiding face-to-face conversations and losing the ability to empathize. She says, "We suppress this capacity by putting ourselves in environments where we're not looking at each other in the eye, not sticking with the other person long enough or hard enough to follow what they're feeling."[29]

> **"We suppress this capacity [for empathy] by putting ourselves in environments where we're not looking at each other in the eye, not sticking with the other person long enough or hard enough to follow what they're feeling."[29]**
>
> —Sherry Turkle is the author of *Reclaiming Conversation: The Power of Talk in the Digital Age.*

The college students Turkle interviewed were positive about the sharing that happens when they brought their cell phones to social interactions. However, Turkle says that "when it came to the bottom-line question, 'What do you think it did to the conversation?' 82 percent say it deteriorated."[30] She also interviewed families about the effect of mobile devices in their communication patterns. She talked to

VIEWPOINT

Cell Phones Are a Distraction in the Classroom

One of the most active debates in education today is the role of cell phones in the classroom. Some educators have reason to ban cell phones. A 2015 study of ninety-one secondary schools in England found that test scores were more than 6 percent higher when cell phones were banned. The improvement was even higher for low-achieving students.

> **This effect is driven by the most disadvantaged and underachieving pupils. Students in the lowest quartile of prior achievement gain 14.23% of a standard deviation, whilst students in the top quartile are neither positively nor negatively affected by a phone ban. The results suggest that low-achieving students are more likely to be distracted by the presence of mobile phones, while high achievers can focus in the classroom regardless of the mobile phone policy.**

Louis-Philippe Beland, "Ill Communication: Technology, Distraction & Student Performance," Centre for Economic Performance, London School of Economics and Political Science, May 2015. http://cep.lse.ac.uk.

three hundred children and teens and found that it was the children who complained about the obsessive use of cell phones by their parents. Thus, in Turkle's view, mobile devices intruded on everyone's ability to sustain face-to-face conversations.

Turkle is not the only researcher who is concerned about the impact of mobile device dependency on human interaction. In a 2014 study titled "The iPhone Effect," researchers listened in on conversations at cafes in Washington, DC, and its surrounding areas. In some instances the pairs of people chatted with a cell phone within eyesight. In other conversations phones were out of sight. The researchers rated each conversation, measuring levels of empathetic concern through various scales. They found that the phones' presence lowered the level of empathy:

> Conversations in the absence of mobile communication technologies were rated as significantly superior compared

with those in the presence of a mobile device, above and beyond the effects of age, gender, ethnicity, and mood. People who had conversations in the absence of mobile devices reported higher levels of empathetic concern. Participants conversing in the presence of a mobile device who also had a close relationship with each other reported lower levels of empathy compared with dyads [pairs] who were less friendly with each other.[31]

In discussions of this study, some experts have suggested that having a cell phone present reminds people that there is a wider world with which they could connect, which may prevent those people from connecting with others right next to them.

VIEWPOINT

Cell Phones Can Have a Positive Impact in Classrooms

Many educators think that because smartphones are connected to the Internet, they can be a powerful aid to student learning. They believe that the way to integrate mobile technology into the classroom is through teacher training. Teacher Carla Dolman, whose Saskatchewan, Canada, school experimented with using cell phones, had positive results. She says:

> **It's a stereotype of teenagers—that you can't trust them with a cell phone. Our experience was that if you give them the opportunity to use them, and you give them guidelines to go with that use, you won't have problems. The more we discover what we can do with them, the more valuable they are. If you can harness what students are interested in, you have massive amounts of potential. And if you can get that into the classroom, you're set.**

Quoted in David Rapp, "Lift the Cell Phone Ban," *Scholastic Administrator*, 2016. www.scholastic.com.

Dependency Reflects Larger Mental Health Issues

Although some researchers operate under the belief that nomophobia and dependency are modern concerns that should be addressed, other experts maintain that most people's use of mobile devices is not as widely problematic or worrisome as critics charge. Dr. Mark Griffiths, director of the International Gaming Research Unit at Nottingham Trent University in the United Kingdom, says that "even though people may be using their smartphones a lot, it's generally life-enhancing. But there will always be a small minority, with any technological advancement, that do it to excess and it causes them problems."[32] He believes that people who compulsively check their phones and whose lives are significantly disrupted by them have underlying mental health issues: "Therapeutically, if you find out what that problem is, then the excessive use can disappear."[33]

A number of experts believe that compulsive mobile device checking is a symptom of an underlying psychological problem such as anxiety or depression. Here, a teenage girl waits anxiously for a reply to a text.

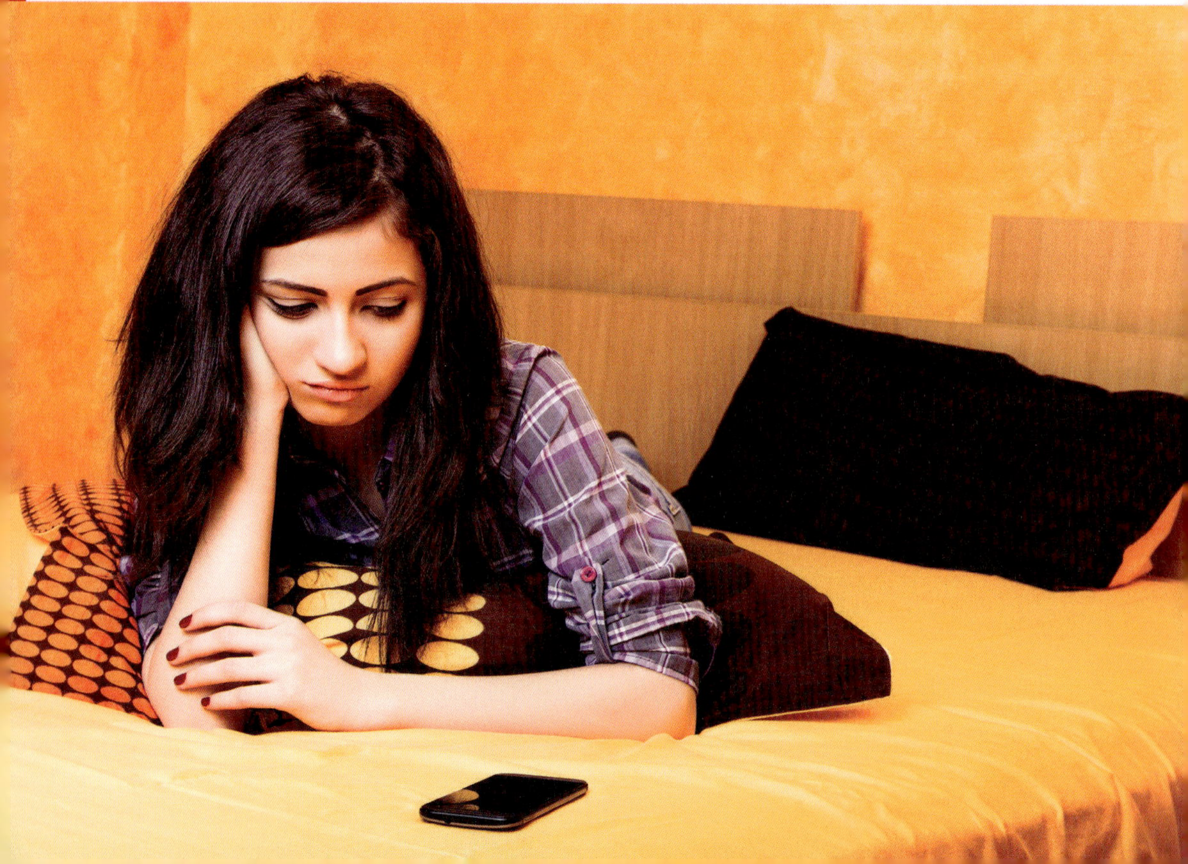

Dr. Lisa Merlo, an assistant professor of psychiatry at the University of Florida College of Medicine, agrees. "When (cell phone overuse) really becomes problematic for a lot of people is if they have underlying anxiety or depression,"[34] she says. For instance, people who worry excessively about how they are perceived by others can become anxious if their phone calls or texts are not immediately answered. People who are depressed may use their phones to distract themselves from a negative mood. Getting professional treatment can allow the sufferers to find more effective ways to cope with their disorder. Thus, compulsive mobile device checking is, for some users, a symptom of personal anxieties and not the sign of a larger social problem.

> **"The evidence consistently shows that the more you communicate with people using devices, the more likely you are to communicate with those people face to face."[35]**
>
> —Nancy Baym is a researcher at Microsoft Research.

The Possibilities of Digital Connections

Nancy Baym, a researcher at Microsoft Research, makes claims similar to those of Griffiths and Merlo. She counters many of the concerns about cell phone dependency with arguments pointing out the positive aspects of mobile devices. In her 2010 book *Personal Connections in the Digital Age*, she challenges the perception that cell phone addiction prevents people from developing healthy relationships. According to Baym, people who access the Internet frequently are more likely to meet with friends, know their neighbors, and spend more time at social occasions. She believes that digital communications enhance relationships and that "the evidence consistently shows that the more you communicate with people using devices, the more likely you are to communicate with those people face to face."[35] She also disputes the argument that texting and e-mailing make it difficult to experience emotion by noting people's innovation in using punctuation, capitalization, and emojis to convey feeling.

App developer Gabriel is also optimistic that people can resist a dependence on smartphones and the constant flow of information they provide. "Millennials are most strongly tied to their smartphones and purport to be less affected by information overload compared to older generations who were not born into the mobile era," he says. He is one of many working for a better understanding of the impact of mobile devices. "For some people, they may just need to understand better how much of their time they are losing to consumption of 'junk food' information. For others, we need clear, forceful evidence—a better understanding of the negative effects of information overindulgence on the brain and pleasure centers."[36]

5 CHAPTER Do Mobile Devices Promote Oversharing?

The *DigiDimwits* video, featuring a blocky animated married couple, is meant to spoof life in the digital age. The husband tells his wife he just posted details of their upcoming vacation to France to his Facebook account. She responds by saying she also put a notice about the vacation in the local newspaper. Incredulous, he asks why she would broadcast such information for the creepy neighbors to know. She replies, "My mistake will only be seen by a few people in town. You gave billions of people a crystal ball into our future."[37] She ends by reminding viewers that what is posted online is public and permanent.

The *Webster's New World Dictionary* word of the year for 2008 was *overshare*. It was defined as "to divulge excessive personal information, as in a blog or broadcast interview, prompting reactions ranging from alarmed discomfort to approval."[38] One of the dictionary's editors explained that some people use the word in a negative way because they do not like oversharing. But he also remarks that "others think oversharing is good and that one must give full disclosure of one's inner life. Sometimes there is a generational shift in the way people look at this practice and therefore view the word. We found that very interesting."[39]

Both the *DigiDimwits* video and the use of the word *overshare* are definitive products of a modern Internet culture. Until the advent of social networking via computer, people exchanged personal information with just a small circle of family members, neighbors, and close friends. As technology has become more sophisticated, opportunities to broadcast details about one's life have expanded exponentially. Because of convenient connected mobile devices, people are sharing more and more information about themselves online. One can snap a photo and have it instantly available to dozens, or in the case of celebrities, millions of friends and followers. The line between sharing and oversharing is shifting.

Why Do People Overshare?

While most people use social media responsibly, some people consistently engage in posting TMI—too much information. Social scientists have put forward many theories for this behavior. In 2012 Harvard researchers, using imaging technology, found that disclosing information about oneself is intrinsically rewarding. Sharing personal emotions, opinions, and images stimulates the brain's pleasure systems. It just feels good. Social media networks allow people to engage in these pleasures by making them feel accepted, especially when others respond to these comments and photos. Status updates and tweets let people share their lives with others.

Canadian researcher Russell W. Belk suggests that some people overshare to become more popular. They can create a better version of themselves. He says that "when we're looking at the screen we're not face-to-face with someone who can immediately respond to us, so it's easier to let it all out—it's almost like we're invisible."[40] *Wall Street Journal* writer Elizabeth Bernstein agrees that popularity is one reason why people overshare. However, she claims that in some instances, it is fans wanting to imitate media culture in which celebrities routinely share the most intimate details of their private lives. On the other hand, Bernstein states that oversharing also happens when people are trying to control their anxiety. She explains that people use up mental energy trying to manage the impression other people have of them. She says, "We try to look smart, witty and interesting, but the effort required to do this leaves less brain power to filter what we say and to whom."[41] She suggests that when people are emotionally exhausted, they let down their guard and often say too much.

> **"When we're looking at the screen we're not face-to-face with someone who can immediately respond to us, so it's easier to let it all out—it's almost like we're invisible."[40]**
>
> —Russell W. Belk is a professor of marketing at York University in Toronto, Canada.

How Do People Overshare?

Facilitating this desire to overshare is a host of platforms designed to post one's thoughts and images. Readers only have to count

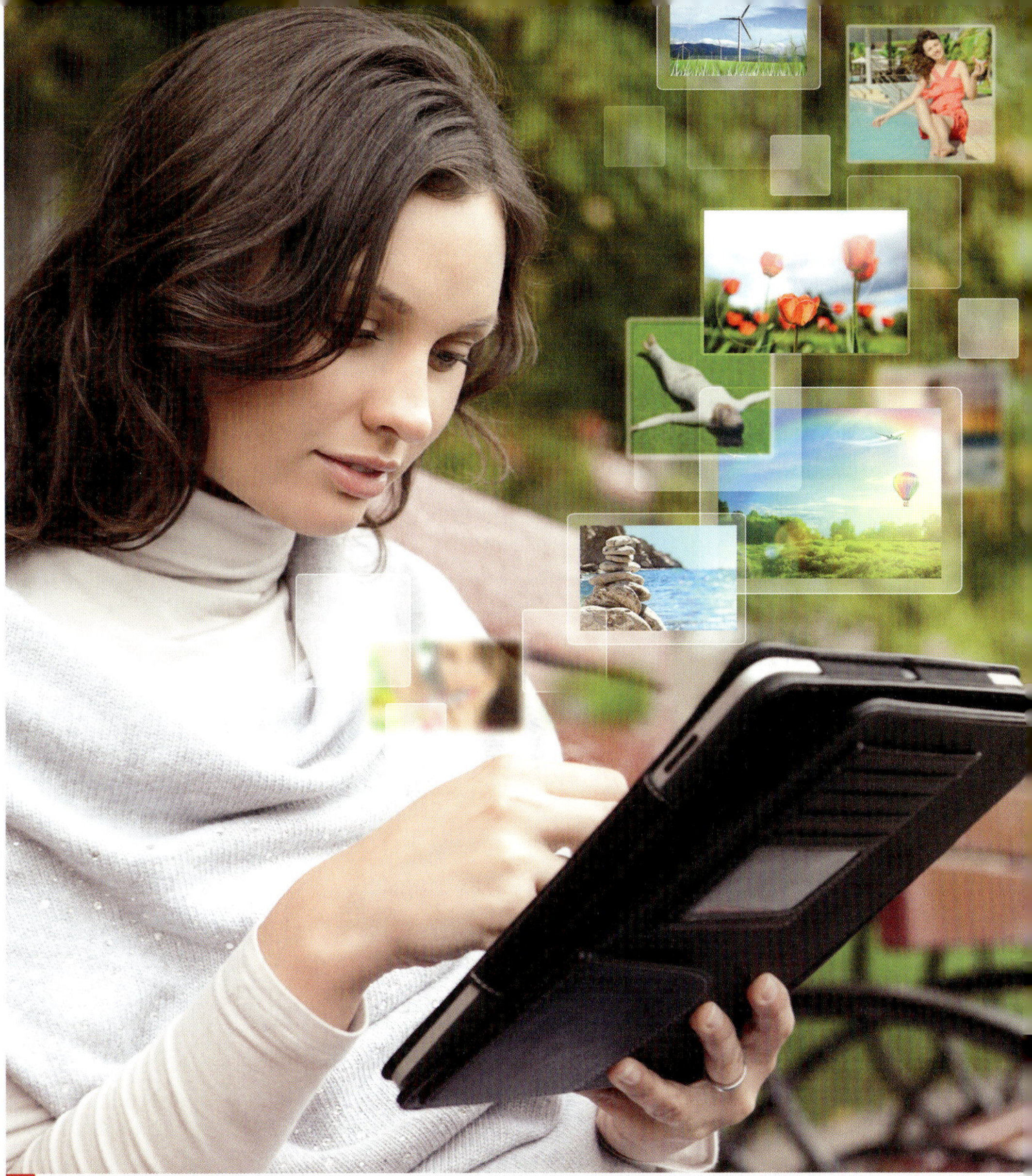

Millions of people enjoy sharing photos and other information about themselves on social media. Some of them, however, consistently engage in posting too much information—a potentially problematic habit known as oversharing.

the number of icons at the top of any news article to see the many ways they can quickly share it with friends. App developers are constantly coming up with new ways for people, especially media-savvy teens, to connect with others to share secrets, follow a crush, or post a selfie. And the variety of social networking sites allows young people to create and experiment with several

VIEWPOINT

Social Media Posts Are Permanent

Many technology experts warn Internet users that everything they post is impossible to delete and will stay online forever. One of these is Eric Tornoe, a computer security expert at the University of St. Thomas is St. Paul, Minnesota. He warns users that deleting a photo or post from social media does not mean that the material is gone. He says:

> **Most of the stuff on the web is living on a hard drive somewhere, and it doesn't cost a whole lot to store. It's nearly impossible to get rid of and it stays there forever. When you erase a disk drive that data is still almost as easy to get back as it is if you haven't erased the drive. [Experts] don't consider anything truly secure unless you physically destroy the drive. Think of your path on the Internet as leaving a permanent footprint. No matter where you go or what you delete, no matter how often you clear your search history, someone with computer expertise can track that footprint through a log of activity.**

Nichelle Heu, "Permanent Footprint," ThreeSixty, September–October 2013. www.threesixty journalism.org.

online profiles. The Pew Research Center reports that 71 percent of teens use more than one social network site. Because of the variety and the options, texting, sharing photos and videos, and meeting new people in cyberspace has never been easier

Most mobile device users choose apps that best fit their needs of the moment. For example, many teens and young adults are flocking to apps that let them communicate anonymously. These sites do allow users to express themselves freely. However, anonymous apps can encourage bullying and inappropriate behavior. Online safety experts warn that anonymous social media sites often become a haven for cyberbullies, who can target their victims without the fear of being discovered. One example is Ask.fm, which lets users ask questions and answer those posted by others. While some are innocent, the site also attracts mean and insulting responses. Kik Messenger is another popular app because users can send unlimited individual or group messages. Common Sense Media rates the app as appropriate for ages seventeen and up due to its pervasive use for sexual content. Both Ask.fm and Kik have been implicated in recent years in high-profile cases of bullying that led to teen suicides. Richard Piggin, deputy chief executive of the charity BeatBullying, called Ask.fm a "stalker's paradise." According to Piggin, "The tool that enables it to be anonymous can facilitate young people to say things that they might not say face to face or if their names were attached to it. So it releases their inhibitions, which can be very dangerous. Sites like Ask.fm lack even the most basic child safety mechanisms. They are of huge concern to us and the young people we work with."[42]

"Sites like Ask.fm lack even the most basic child safety mechanisms. They are of huge concern to us and the young people we work with."[42]

—Richard Piggin is the deputy chief executive of the charity BeatBullying.

VIEWPOINT

Interest in Social Media Posts Is Not Permanent

Some experts disagree with warnings that once a photo is posted on social media, it will circulate forever. Anthony Rotolo, a professor of social media at Syracuse University, finds that older material loses its appeal and does eventually disappear from Internet searches. He says:

> There's a half life to the stuff that we share online, and it's really short. The Internet lives on moments. It lives on what is viral right now, whether globally (like Justin Bieber getting arrested), or viral within your own social network. Then it's over very quickly. What we're seeing is that your naked pictures from 10 years ago are nowhere near as appealing as someone else's new naked pictures, which will be forgotten tomorrow anyway.

Quoted in Patrick Di Justo, "Naked on the Internet Is Not Forever," *Atlantic*, February 7, 2014. www.theatlantic.com.

Colleges Check Social Media

Oversharing can cause unintended consequences for teens who are not yet thinking beyond the drama of high school. According to the *New York Times*, one high school senior found out the hard way that colleges care about the social media presence of their students. All through Bowdoin College's informational presentation for prospective students, the young woman tweeted insulting remarks to her friends about the other students attending the presentation. Like most colleges, Bowdoin tracks its social media mentions. Therefore, the young woman was denied admission. "We would have wondered about the judgment of someone who spends their time on their mobile phone and makes such awful remarks,"[43] Bowdoin's dean of admissions told reporter Natasha Singer.

Test preparation company Kaplan found that 30 percent of colleges visit applicants' social media accounts, and about 30 percent of them find information that reflects negatively on the students. For instance, in 2012 a Pitzer College undergraduate in Claremont, California, friended a prospective student on Facebook. The Pitzer undergrad notified college officials when he saw that the prospective student had posted offensive comments about one of the student's high school teachers. The student was not considered for admission.

On the other hand, social media can boost students' chances for admission. Colleges participate in most large social media and microblogging sites, allowing them to interact with potential applicants. On these sites, students can highlight accomplishments in writing, music, athletics, animation, entrepreneurship, fashion, dance, and drama. Today's digital natives are adept at making and posting sophisticated videos that showcase their skills and talents.

Oversharing Can Impact Employment

It is not just higher education that investigates the social media content of applicants. When employers hire new employees, they make a significant investment in their new hires. Hiring managers want to find out as much about job applicants as they can before offering someone a job. But employers are limited by what appli-

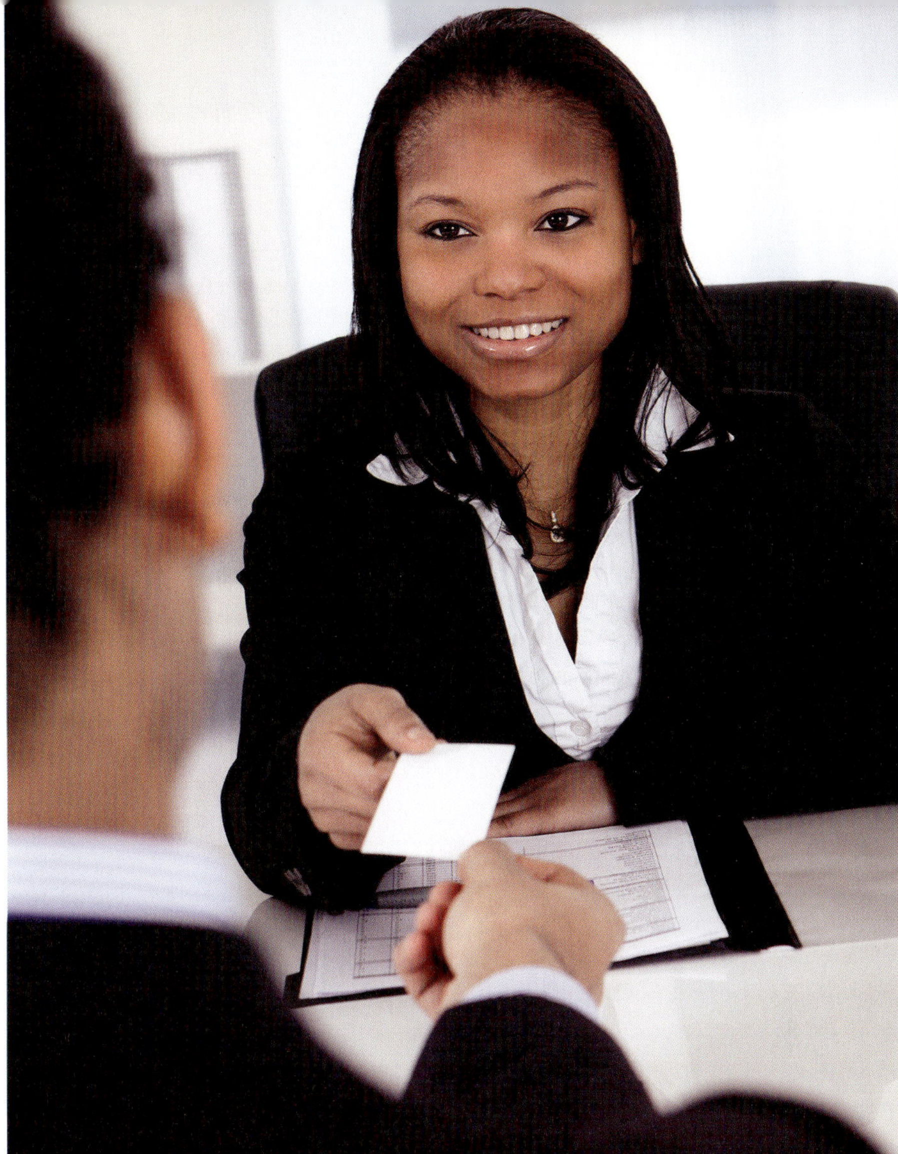

A recruiter interviews a job candidate. Increasingly, employers are rejecting job applicants who have used social media to post questionable content about themselves, such as sexually explicit images or photos of illicit drug use.

cants choose to reveal about themselves on their job applications and in interviews. At least, they were until the advent of social media opened a window into people's lives.

Some employers use investigation companies to scour the Internet for information about potential new hires as a sort of social media background check. Investigators sometimes find information that is not relevant to the job but may cause employers to reject the applicant. Max Drucker, CEO of Internet security company Social Intelligence, tells of one company that rejected an applicant because he used Craigslist to look for painkillers. Employers passed on another applicant who posted nude photos of herself on Instagram. According to Drucker, it is photos and videos taken impulsively on mobile devices that get people into the most trouble. "Sexually explicit photos and videos are beyond comprehension," he says. "We also see flagrant displays of weapons. And we see a lot of illegal activity. Lots and lots of pictures of drug use."[44] According to Drucker, 70 percent of job recruiters report that they have rejected applicants because of what they had posted online.

Smart mobile device users, however, can use their social media accounts to impress potential employers. Photos posted to Facebook, Instagram, or Tumblr that show past achievements in school or extracurricular activities provide evidence of teamwork skills and a strong work ethic. Facebook users can transfer their networking skills to LinkedIn and make valuable connections to leaders who can help with job and career moves.

Children's and Teens' Privacy Can Be Compromised

Another group of mobile device users who overshare are parents who post photos of their children on social media sites. By making the photos available for anyone to see, parents unwittingly put their children at risk. The primary risk for the children is identity theft, but other risks include stalking, kidnapping, and molestation. In a 2015 study titled "Children Seen but Not Heard: When Parents Compromise Children's Online Privacy," a research team combed through social media to find parents who had posted photos of children in one East Coast town. The team combined the parents' social media profile data with public voter registration records and found the parents' home addresses. Using easily available facial recognition software and comments and tags on children's photos, they were able to deduce the children's full names, addresses, and birthdays. Tehila Minkus, lead author of the study, states that its purpose "was not to publicly expose sensitive information about children, but rather to raise public awareness about the results of oversharing."[45] One result, she points out, is that the public information prevents children from hiding their online presences if they later wish to do so. Another concern is that the public information makes it easier for identity thieves to acquire a child's Social Security number. In addition, children's privacy, financial reputation, and credit history can become compromised before they become an adult.

The online privacy study's authors made several recommendations to safeguard the privacy of minors. They advised parents to make Facebook and Instagram private so that only approved friends and followers can see photos. Parents should avoid tagging photos with names, birthdays, locations, or any other personal information.

It is not just parents who compromise safety by oversharing on social media. There is evidence that preteens and teens are posting personal information that could put them at risk for bullying, stalking, home burglary, and identity theft. A 2014 study by Internet security company McAfee reported that 39 percent of teens did not adjust their social networking profiles to protect their content. Fifty percent of teens posted their e-mail address, 30 percent their phone number, and 14 percent their home address. All of these behaviors allow teens' locations to be visible to acquaintances and strangers who might want to harass or stalk them. Some teens, excited to get their first bank debit card, have even posted a photo of it to social media. This readily available online data leaves teens vulnerable to identity theft.

Oversharing Can Lead to Sexting

Identity theft is not the only Internet-related crime that teens need to be concerned about. Many teens do not realize that sending and receiving sexually explicit photos can be a crime. A combination of the words *sex* and *texting*, sexting is sending or receiving a photo of someone engaged in a sexual act, posed in a sexually explicit manner, or otherwise sexually excited. Sexting also includes sending sexually explicit messages, voice mails, and videos. According to a 2014 Drexel University study, more than 50 percent of teens have sent or received sexually explicit

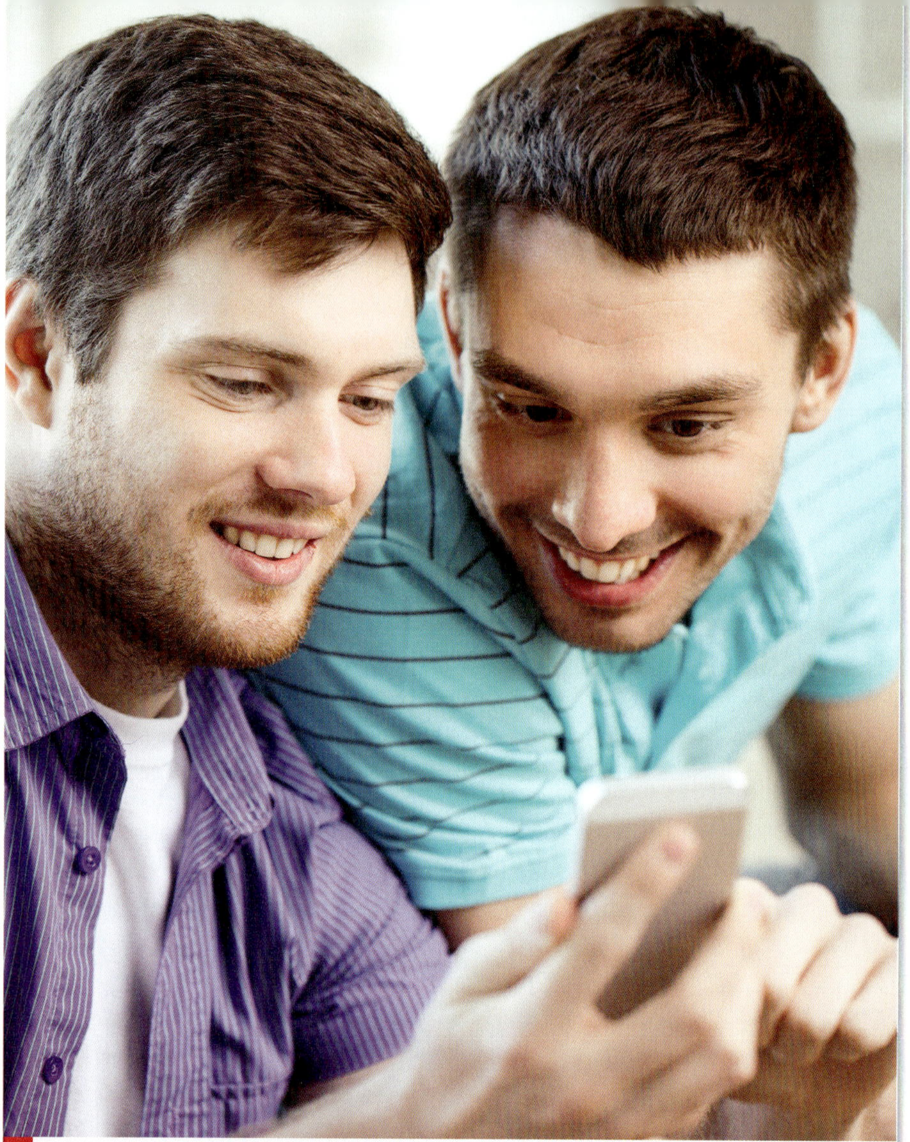

Young men look at images on a smartphone. Teens who engage in sexting, or sending sexually explicit images of themselves to others via a mobile device, often find that something they intended solely for one person has instead been shared with multiple people.

messages, 20 percent have sent or received sexually provocative messages, and 25 percent have sent or received nude or semi-nude photos. Some teens send sexts to attract the attention of a potential boyfriend or girlfriend. Others want to increase their popularity by looking "hot."

Sexting can quickly get out of hand. Teens sometimes send photos to friends that show them in compromising situations, thinking their friends will keep them private. Internet security expert Steve Woda warns teens that their friends

> may not be the best decision makers when it comes to protecting personal info. The ease of re-sharing digital messages or photos puts the decision making power in the hands of the recipient, who may not think twice about sending it to others. Once the personal information (intended for certain recipients) leaves the circle of trust, it can spread through the community like a wildfire.[46]

Sexting can have serious consequences. In many communities, a teen who sends or receives a sexually explicit photo can be charged with promoting, distributing, and possessing child pornography. In 2016 five Newtown, Connecticut, high school students were arrested for sexting, and twenty more were referred to a juvenile review board. Some of the students were charging money for the photos. They were using smartphone apps such as Snapchat, FaceTime, iMessage, and Kik. State laws have not kept up with current technology when it comes to sending or receiving nude photos by a minor. Teens who are caught are often prosecuted under felony child pornography or child exploitation laws. Teens who are convicted may go to jail and have to register as a sex offender for the rest of their lives. However, some critics consider this punishment too severe for adolescents who are beginning to explore their sexuality. In most cases the teens do not realize they may be breaking any laws. States such as Arizona, Hawaii, Nevada, and New York have rewritten their laws and consider sending sexually explicit messages or photos by people under the age of eighteen a petty offense punishable by a fine or community service. Teens who receive sexually explicit material

"[Friends] may not be the best decision makers when it comes to protecting personal info. The ease of re-sharing digital messages or photos puts the decision making power in the hands of the recipient, who may not think twice about sending it to others."[46]

—Steve Woda is the president and CEO of uKnow, which creates Internet safety products.

without requesting it and immediately delete it incur no legal consequences. Numerous other states are considering revising their sexting laws.

Not everyone thinks sexting is out-of-control criminal behavior. Some psychologists find sexual exploration normal among adolescents. They consider sexting as a contemporary form of intimate communication between romantic partners. They say that teens are imitating the adult behaviors they see in the celebrities they admire. One expert advises school officials to stop demonizing what she considers a part of teens' sexual development. Psychologist Elizabeth Englander, director of the Massachusetts Aggression Reduction Center at Bridgewater State University, says that despite recent high-profile media attention, she found few psychological problems associated with sexting. According to Englander, "When I studied the after effects of sexting, I found that most incidents didn't have much of an outcome at all—either good or bad. Most kids didn't describe trauma or bullying, but neither did they describe newly-acquired boyfriends or increased popularity. The most common outcome was generally 'feeling worse,' but even that happened in only about one-quarter of the cases."[47]

"When I studied the after effects of sexting, I found that most incidents didn't have much of an outcome at all—either good or bad. Most kids didn't describe trauma or bullying, but neither did they describe newly-acquired boyfriends or increased popularity."[47]

—Elizabeth Englander is director of the Massachusetts Aggression Reduction Center at Bridgewater State University.

Technology experts and social science researchers agree that mobile devices have made oversharing personal details about one's life easy and prevalent. Though they warn about the dangers of oversharing, they are optimistic that through awareness and education, mobile device users—especially teens and young adults—can learn to set clear boundaries between what is fun and beneficial and what is damaging. Mobile devices are a necessity in today's world and are an integral part of modern life. Cell phones do have the potential to cause harm to the people who use them. However, experts are confident that mobile device users can make good choices once they have a clear understanding of the consequences of their actions.

Introduction: A Deadly Crash

1. Quoted in Matt Richtel, *A Deadly Wandering*. New York: Morrow, 2014, p. 91.
2. Quoted in Richtel, *A Deadly Wandering*, p. 146.
3. Quoted in Richtel, *A Deadly Wandering*, p. 303.

Chapter 1: What Are The Facts?

4. Quoted in Zachary Davies Boren, "There Are Officially More Mobile Devices in the World than People," *Independent* (London), October 7, 2014. www.independent.co.uk.
5. Amanda Lenhart, "Teens, Social Media & Technology Overview 2015," Pew Research Center, April 9, 2015. www.pewinternet.org.
6. Howard Gardner and Katie Davis, *The App Generation*. New Haven, CT: Yale University Press, 2013, p. 7.
7. Instagram, "FAQ," 2016. www.instagram.com.

Chapter 2: Do Mobile Phones Impair Users' Physical Health?

8. Quoted in Norwegian Institute of Public Health, "Mobile Phones and Wireless Networks: No Evidence of Health Risk Found," September 12, 2012. www.fhi.no.
9. Quoted in Brian Farmer, "Scientists Warn Congress of Cellphone Cancer Risk," *New American*, October 1, 2008. www.thenewamerican.com.
10. Luis Landestoy. "Luis Commits to Health, Happiness & UP3," Get Up Together, 2016. http://jawbone.com.
11. Quoted in Olga Khazan, "How Smartphones Hurt Sleep," *Atlantic*, February 24, 2015. www.theatlantic.com.
12. Quoted in Brady Dennis, "iPads, Tablets, Smartphones Disrupt Good Sleep, Study Finds," *Washington Post*, December 22, 2014. www.washingtonpost.com.
13. Quoted in *Sleep Review*, "Cell Phone Addicts Most Sleep Deprived," November 14, 2014. www.sleepreviewmag.com.

Chapter 3: Are Mobile Devices a Dangerous Distraction?

14. Quoted in Carnegie Mellon University, "Carnegie Mellon Study Provides Conclusive Evidence That Cell Phones Distract Drivers," EurekAlert!, July 26, 2001. www.eurekalert.org.

15. Quoted in Vanderbilt News, "Neural Bottleneck Found That Thwarts Multi-tasking," January 18, 2007. http://news.vanderbilt.edu.
16. David Strayer et al., "Measuring Cognitive Distraction in the Automobile III: A Comparison of Ten 2015 In-Vehicle Information Systems," AAA Foundation for Traffic Safety, October 2015. http://newsroom.aaa.com.
17. Quoted in Wayne State University, "Study by Wayne State University Research Shows Early Studies on Cellphone Conversations Likely Overestimated Crash Risk," December 14, 2011. http://wayne.edu.

Chapter 4: Are People Too Dependent on Mobile Devices?

18. Nala Cheng, "Do You Suffer from Disconnect Anxiety?," Voices of Youth, 2015. www.voicesofyouth.org.
19. Quoted in Stephen Shankland, "Enough, Already! Why We All Share the Blame for Notification Overload," CNET, July 10, 2015. www.cnet.com.
20. Quoted in Shankland, "Enough, Already! Why We All Share the Blame for Notification Overload."
21. Quoted in Tony Gonzalez, "Nashville High Schoolers Give Up Phones for a Day—See How They Survived," Nashville Public Radio, November 2, 2015. http://nashvillepublicradio.org.
22. Quoted in Gonzalez, "Nashville High Schoolers Give Up Phones for a Day—See How They Survived."
23. Nancy Jo Sales, *American Girls: Social Media and the Secret Lives of Teenagers*. New York: Knopf, 2016, p. 10.
24. *The World UNPLUGGED* (blog), "Going 24 Hours Without Media," 2010. http://theworldunplugged.wordpress.com.
25. Quoted in *The World UNPLUGGED* (blog), "Going 24 Hours Without Media."
26. Quoted in Lulu Chang, "Addicted to Your Smartphone. This App Developer Explains Why," Digital Trends, January 24, 2016. www.digitaltrends.com.
27. Quoted in Nara Schoenberg, "Is Your Smartphone Hurting Your GPA?," *Chicago Tribune*, March 6, 2013. http://articles.chicagotribune.com.
28. Cary Stothart et al., "The Attentional Cost of Receiving a Cell Phone Notification," *Journal of Experimental Psychology: Human Perception and Performance*, pp. 893–897, June 29, 2015.

29. Quoted in Lauren Cassani Davis, "The Flight from Conversation," *Atlantic*, October 7, 2015. www.theatlantic.com.
30. Quoted in Davis, "The Flight from Conversation."
31. Shalini Misra et al., "The iPhone Effect: The Quality of In-Person Social Interactions in the Presence of Mobile Devices," *Environment and Behavior*, July 1, 2014. http://eab.sagepub.com.
32. Quoted in Simon Hill, "Is Smartphone Addiction Real? We Ask the Experts," Digital Trends, November 1, 2015. www.digitaltrends.com.
33. Quoted in Hill, "Is Smartphone Addiction Real? We Ask the Experts."
34. Quoted in UF News, "Addicted to Phones? Cell Phone Use Becoming a Major Problem for Some, Expert Says," January 18, 2007. http://news.ufl.edu.
35. Quoted in Iris Adler, "How Our Digital Devices Are Affecting Our Personal Relationships," WBUR, January 17, 2013. www.wbur.org.
36. Quoted in Chang, "Addicted to Your Smartphone. This App Developer Explains Why."

Chapter 5: Do Mobile Devices Promote Oversharing?

37. *The DigiDimwits*, video, Internet Safety Source, 2015. www.internetsafetysource.com.
38. *Webster's New World* (blog), "Word of the Year," 2008. http://wordoftheyear.wordpress.com.
39. Quoted in *Webster's New World* (blog), "Word of the Year."
40. Quoted in Paul Hiebert, "The Real Reason Why So Many People Overshare on Facebook," *Slate*, August 19, 2013. www.slate.com.
41. Quoted in Hiebert, "The Real Reason Why So Many People Overshare on Facebook."
42. Quoted in NoBullying.com, "Understanding the Reasons Behind Ask.fm Bullying," September 25, 2014. http://nobullying.com.
43. Quoted in Natasha Singer, "They Loved Your G.P.A. Then They Saw Your Tweets," *New York Times*, November 9, 2013. www.nytimes.com.

44. Quoted in Jennifer Preston, "Social Media History Becomes a New Job Hurdle," *New York Times*, July 20, 2011. www.nytimes.com.
45. Tehila Minkus et al., "Children Seen but Not Heard: When Parents Compromise Children's Online Privacy," International World Wide Web Conference Committee, 2015. http://cse.poly.edu.
46. Steve Woda, "Oversharing Online: How One Post Can Damage Your Kid's Reputation," uKnowKids, August 1, 2014. http://uknowkids.com.
47. Elizabeth Englander, "Stop Demonizing Teen Sexting. In Most Cases It Is Completely Harmless," *Washington Post*, November 7, 2014. www.washingtonpost.com.

Cellular Telecommunications & Internet Association (CTIA)

1400 Sixteenth St. NW, Suite 600
Washington, DC 20036
phone: (202) 736-3200
website: www.ctia.org

The CTIA is an international nonprofit organization whose members include wireless carriers and providers and manufacturers of wireless data services. Its website contains facts and resources about cybersafety and using mobile devices safely while driving.

Common Sense Media

650 Townsend St., Suite 435
San Francisco, CA 94103
phone: (415) 863-0600
website: http://commonsensemedia.org

The mission of Common Sense Media is to empower parents, teachers, and policy makers by providing information, advice, and tools to use media wisely. The agency helps students make smart choices when using digital media.

Distraction.gov

1200 New Jersey Ave. SE, West Building
Washington, DC 20590
phone: (888) 327-4236
website: www.distraction.gov

Distraction.gov is the US Department of Transportation website for information on distracted driving. It contains facts, resources, and legal information about distracted driving.

International Agency for Research on Cancer (IARC)

150 Cours Albert Thomas
69372 Lyon CEDEX 08
France
phone: 33 04 72 73 84 85
website: www.iarc.fr

Part of the World Health Organization, the IARC promotes international collaboration for cancer research, including research that investigates the relationship between mobile devices and various cancers.

Media Smarts

950 Gladstone Ave., Suite 120
Ottawa, ON
Canada K1Y 3E6
phone: (613) 224-7721
website: http://mediasmarts.ca

Media Smarts is a not-for-profit organization that provides digital and media literacy. Its goal is to teach children and teens the critical-thinking skills needed to become active and informed digital citizens.

National Highway Traffic Safety Administration (NHTSA)

1200 New Jersey Ave. SE, West Building
Washington, DC 20590
phone: (888) 327-4236
website: www.nhtsa.gov

The NHTSA is an office of the US Department of Transportation. Its mission is to prevent traffic-related injuries and deaths. It provides resources about distracted driving and the use of mobile devices while driving.

StopBullying.gov

200 Independence Ave. SW
Washington, DC 20201
phone: (877) 696-6775
website: www.stopbullying.gov

StopBullying.gov is a federal government website that explains what bullying is and what children, teens, parents, and educators can do to prevent it. It provides resources to assist teens in dealing with cyberbullying and using technology safely.

World Health Organization (WHO)
Avenue Appia 20
1211 Geneva 27, Switzerland
phone: 41 22 791 21 11
website: www.who.int

WHO provides research and information on issues related to health, including new technologies and mobile devices. Its website provides resources that explain the impact of electromagnetic and radiation emissions on mobile device users.

Books

danah boyd, *It's Complicated: The Social Lives of Networked Teens*. New Haven, CT: Yale University Press, 2014.

Roman Espejo, *Smartphones*. Detroit, MI: Greenhaven, 2013.

Howard Gardner and Katie Davis, *The App Generation*. New Haven, CT: Yale University Press, 2013.

Rebecca T. Klein, *Frequently Asked Questions About Text, Sexting and Flaming*. New York: Rosen, 2013.

Patricia Netzley, *How Do Cell Phones Affect Health?* San Diego: ReferencePoint, 2015.

Larry D. Rosen, *iDisorder: Understanding Our Obsession with Technology and Overcoming Its Hold on Us*. New York: Macmillan, 2012.

Nancy Jo Sales, *American Girls: Social Media and the Secret Lives of Teenagers*. New York: Knopf, 2016.

Catherine Steiner-Adair and Teresa H. Barker, *The Big Disconnect: Protecting Childhood and Family Relationships in the Digital Age*. New York: HarperCollins, 2013.

Sherry Turkle, *Reclaiming Conversation: The Power of Talk in a Digital Age*. New York: Penguin, 2016.

Internet Sources

Devra Davis, "Beyond Brain Cancer: Other Possible Dangers of Cell Phones," *Huffington Post*, June 15, 2011. www.huffingtonpost.com/devra-davis-phd/cell-phones-cancer_b_874361.html.

Mackenzie Dawson, "How Social Media Is Destroying the Lives of Teen Girls," *New York Post*, February 21, 2016. http://nypost.com/2016/02/21/how-social-media-is-destroying-the-lives-of-teen-girls.

Samantha Edwards, "Sexting: The New Normal for Teens," WCSH6-TV, April 24, 2015. http://legacy.wcsh6.com/story/news/local/2015/04/23/sexting-the-new-normal/26240501.

Christine Elgersma, "16 Apps and Websites Kids Are Heading to After Facebook," *Parenting, Media, and Everything in Between* (blog), Common Sense Media, March 1, 2016. www.commonsensemedia.org./blog/16-apps-and-websites-kids-are-heading-to-after-facebook.

Olga Khazan, “How Smartphones Hurt Sleep,” *Atlantic*, February 24, 2015. www.theatlantic.com/health/archive/2015/02/how-smartphones-are-ruining-our-sleep/385792.

David Strayer et al., “Measuring Cognitive Distraction in the Automobile III: A Comparison of Ten 2015 In-Vehicle Information Systems,” AAA Foundation for Traffic Safety, October 2015. https://newsroom.aaa.com/wp-content/uploads/2015/10/Phase-III-Research-Report.pdf.

Marion K. Underwood and Robert W. Faris, “Being 13: Perils of Lurking on Social Media,” CNN, October 6, 2015. http://www.cnn.com/2015/10/05/opinions/underwood-faris-being-thirteen-lurking-social-media/index.html.

Websites

AAA Foundation for Traffic Safety (www.aaafoundation.org). The mission of the AAA Foundation for Traffic Safety is to conduct research to address growing highway safety issues, including distracted driving. It works to identify traffic safety problems, foster research that seeks solutions, and disseminate information and educational materials.

It Can Wait (www.itcanwait.com). It Can Wait is an initiative by major US cell phone carriers that focuses on educating people—especially teens—about the dangers of texting and driving. The website contains educational videos, resources, and statistics.

A Thin Line (www.athinline.org). Developed by MTV, A Thin Line empowers youth to identify, respond to, and stop the spread of digital abuse. It educated teens and young adults about the “thin line” between harmless activities and forced sexting, textual harassment, and cyberbullying.

Wired Safety (www.wiredsafety.org). Wired Safety is an online safety, education, and help group. It provides information and education about safety, privacy, and security issues related to cell phone and other Internet use.

INDEX

Cover: iStockphoto/Daisy-Daisy

6: sjlocke/Depositphotos.com

10: Mactrunk/Depositphotos.com

13: tulpahn/Depositphotos.com

17: Alexey_boldin/Depositphotos.com

22: stockdevil_666/Depositphotos.com

27: urban_light/Depositphotos.com

29: CandyBoxImages/Depositphotos.com

33: sjlocke/Depositphotos.com

37: Syda_Productions/Depositphotos.com

41: londondeposit/Depositphotos.com

44: mantinov/Depositphotos.com

48: photographee.eu/Depositphotos.com

52: jinga80/Depositphotos.com

57: HASLOO/Depositphotos.com

61: AndreyPopov/Depositphotos.com

64: Syda_Productions/Depositphotos.com